ANIMALITY

ANIMALITY

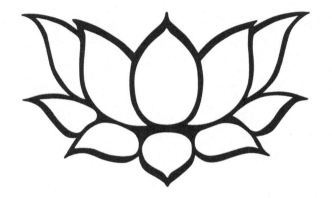

How Pets and People Connect

BY MELISSA L. MAGNUSON, DVM

This book is dedicated to Freckles, Pepper and Sam, my childhood (dog) friends, my pet pig, Turkey, and many named and nameless barn cats.

TABLE OF CONTENTS

INTRODUCTION...1

Chapter 1: BECOMING A VETERNARIAN...6

Chapter 2: ZOOBIQUITY...21

Chapter 3: GESTALT...40

Chapter 4: HOW PETS EXPRESS AFFECTION...51

Chapter 5: TRUST THEIR INSTINCTS...64

Chapter 6: ANIMAL COMMUNICATION..78

Chapter 7: YOUR PET IS YOUR MIRROR...92

Chapter 8: DON'T STRESS THEM OUT...102

Chapter 9: COMMON SENSE FROM THE CONSCIOUS VET....................120

Chapter 10: MIRACLE STORIES..127

Chapter 11: SAYING GOODBYE...140

AFTERWORD...147

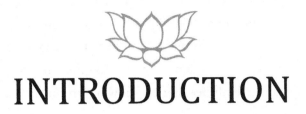

INTRODUCTION

If there is one given in my life it's this: I find animals that are in need of care. Whether they are sick, hurt or lost, I find them.

Or maybe it's the other way around. Animals always find me.

Growing up on a farm gave me plenty of opportunity to make friends with all kinds of animals including cats, dogs, horses, chickens, pigs and cows. I spent much of my time outside and in the animal barns where we raised cattle and pigs to be sold as our livelihood. As a child, I really didn't understand the business part. I thought the animals were there for me to talk to each day. We bonded.

One of my jobs was to give the baby pigs iron injections. Shortly after baby pigs were born, they would need an iron shot to help them grow. The pig barns were filled with hundreds of pigs of all different ages and sizes. I would also identify the "runts" or small ones and keep an eye on them to make sure they were nursing because they would often be pushed away by the other bigger baby pigs.

I was especially drawn to the little ones, maybe because they were so small or maybe because they just drew me in. Out of the hundreds of pigs in my care, one such runt was extra tiny and extra needy. I connected with him.

I named him Turkey.

Since Turkey was so small, I decided it would be a good idea to bottle-feed him three times a day so he would have a better chance at survival. I would bring the bottle of milk replacer out to the barn every morning, afternoon and evening to feed Turkey. Soon, I did not need to go to the barn, Turkey would come find me. He was so small that he would fit between the slats in the pen and escape the big barn. It became a joyous routine. He would seek me out every morning for his early feeding by showing up on the back step of the house.

"Here Turkey, Turkey, Turkey!" I'd yell.

And a pig would come running.

One morning, I overslept, which was unlike me. I was taught to be extremely responsible from a very young age. My father would have no tolerance for me missing my chores because of sleep. I begged my mother to feed Turkey that morning, so I wouldn't miss the school bus and she agreed. I told her to go out on the back step with the bottle of milk replacer and yell, "Here Turkey, Turkey, Turkey."

Now, my mother was not much of an animal person and she particularly did not like cats. I would even say that she hated cats. She especially hated them weaving in and out of legs and rubbing up on her. She also hated participating in any "animal activities" and stayed in the house most of the time. Now, every morning when I would go outside to do chores, all the barn cats would come running because they knew I would feed them. When I say all, I mean about 15 to 20 cats swarming me and weaving in and out of my legs. It was such chaos that you could barely walk to the barn to feed them.

This morning was no different. After my mother yelled for Turkey the pig, 15 to 20 barn cats crowded her legs and surrounded her. She became very annoyed and was going to go inside, but then she noticed a very small pig in the sea of cats.

"By God, that kid was right," she said. "It's a pig!"

It was not just any pig, but my pet pig, Turkey. Every other day, I was with that pig…connected.

Like I said.

Animals find me.

I find them.

It's not just my job. It's my life.

New Hampshire is known for its Nor'easters, winter storms that occur along the Eastern Seaboard and are famous for their excessive winds and large amounts of snowfall. Even when there are Nor'easters, my animal hospitals stay open because there are always sick animals that need help.

One particular Nor'easter morning, I was navigating the slippery back roads of my hometown on the way to treat a few patients. As a veterinarian who tries to be on time, I'll often take the back roads to avoid New England traffic.

That crazy, snowy day, it wasn't the other cars slowing me down, but the weather. There I was inching along on my way to work in the storm when I saw something strange in the road and gingerly pumped the brakes. As I approached, I was rather shocked to see a formidable bird located in front of my vehicle.

There was a rooster standing in the middle of the road.

I stopped my truck, climbed out into the storm and locked eyes with this bird that was just standing there in the danger zone in more ways than one. The little fellow could have easily been hit, and given the fact that the temperature had sunk to the low teens, it could have also frozen to death.

A quick glance and I knew that the bird's comb – the fleshy growth or crest on top of the head of turkeys, pheasants and chickens, or in this case, a rooster – was frostbitten.

Standing in the road a foot away from another unlikely patient, I knew I couldn't reason with this victim of winter or say, "Just stand there and I'll pick you up. Literally."

The great thing about animals, however, is they have an innate knowing when someone is there to help and most will surrender. Mr. Rooster stood still while I gently approached him and scooped him up in my parka-covered arms.

Where does one put a rooster in a truck? Well, he sat quite nicely in the seat next to me, a very civil travel companion that had an air about him like he was supposed to be there.

A few staff members at my veterinary hospital were a little surprised when I rushed in and immediately put him on a treatment table. Shrugging off my coat, it went like this: "What are you doing?" one asked.

"Oh, I found him in the middle of the road," I said.

"You found a rooster? In the middle of the road in a Nor'easter? Only you would find a rooster!"

Maybe this is why I like to call myself the Conscious Vet.

On my watch, I'd like to think no animal is left behind.

I don't want to keep you in suspense. I warmed up my new rooster friend, treated his frostbite and smiled when he started *cock-a-doodle-doo-ing* loud enough to be heard in our front office.

"Um, Dr. Magnuson, we can't just *keep* a rooster here," said one staff member who thought to bring logic into it. "He's cute, but he's also sort of loud and disruptive. And there are two poodles in the corner that are shaking because apparently they're not big rooster fans."

What does one do with a homeless rooster? Well, I found him a local farm that really needed a rooster and my now-healthy bird sat down (again) in the passenger side of my truck when I drove him to his new home. I've done the same for countless cats and dogs because we are all beings on one planet.

We all deserve a home, food, water and unconditional love. This makes for a peaceful life. This is how animals work. They find us.

Why not lend a hand? It's part of my animal nature or animality to tend to others, plus I find nothing more rewarding.

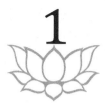

1

Becoming A Veterinarian

Now that we've covered the plight of misfortunate pigs and half frozen roosters, I wanted to introduce myself.

I'm Dr. Melissa Magnuson, DVM, wife to my best friend Andy, mom of three beautiful daughters …and four dogs, a cat, a Meyers parrot, a bearded dragon and a guinea pig.

The idea to become a veterinarian began when I was two-years-old and growing up on a small pig and cattle farm in southern Minnesota. I always joke (although this is actually true) that there were only two people who came to visit our farm, which was 20 miles from town: One was the milkman; the other was far more thrilling for me. Yes, it was the veterinarian.

I liked to drink my milk, but I was absolutely in love with what the vet did when he visited. First of all, he had the coolest truck and all these fun things on it to help our cattle and pigs stay healthy. Despite the fact that I was just a little girl, he allowed me to help him dehorn the cattle or treat a sick horse or pig. No one thought that a small child helping the animals was a bit out of the ordinary since I come from a long line of farmers who rely on the entire family to make sure things run smoothly.

The only thing missing for an animal person such as myself was my own house dog or cat to curl up with at night. Sadly, my sister had severe allergies to the point where she couldn't even go into the barns without getting really sick. Her chores were to clean the house and do the dishes. Meanwhile, I was tasked to work in the barns where I would give pigs iron injections and feed the baby animals.

It was all in a day's work on the farm.

Healing gave me the most joy, especially if I could do anything to alleviate the pain or stress for even one of the animals.

For a split-second, I thought about becoming a people doctor because the idea of healing humans was appealing, too. My biology teacher during my junior year of high school even made a science type like me take an EMT class. Quickly, I learned that I didn't want to do human medicine. I'm very empathic and when people are injured and hurting, it pains me to the core. With animals, I felt their spirits and could be empathetic and understanding when it came to their pain, but I could also separate myself more to make better decisions for them.

I lost my heart to my animals. You could say I fell hard.

Growing up, we had a lot of barn cats, but could never afford to spay and neuter all of them. In fact, we could never spend money on a cat because our budget didn't stretch that far. Sadly, distemper virus would kill a lot of my furry, four-legged barn friends. I did what I could to help the mama cats when they gave birth to kittens and watched them make their nests between bales of straw.

I'll never forget reaching my hands into the nest and counting how many kittens were born. I could feel each little life, soft and silky fur on my fingers contrasting with the prickly straw on the sides. I would touch each and every one of them, doing my counts to see how may new babies there were. Some would live; some would not. I always knew which ones would die because I'd hold the newborn kitten in my palm on its back. If they could hold their head up, they would live. If the head flopped, the kitten would die. I'd try everything possible to help the floppy ones including hand feeding them. I tried to figure out why this was happening and wanted to make a vaccine to prevent this in the future. I even had a special pet cemetery to bury the ones that didn't live and give them a small funeral where I'd say a few kind words about their short existences. Every life mattered.

It was a bit of a lonely life living on a farm and I found out at an early age that animals of all shapes and sizes provided friendship and unconditional love. They are always present, always with you in the moment and they are quite mindful. Later, I'd learn that without putting it into those words, these are the types of connections many people share with their pets.

In fact, in my 20 plus years as a veterinarian, the statement that resonates with me the most is when someone says to me, "You have no idea what my pet means to me."

I tell them, "I do… I do know."

When I was twelve, I begged my father for a Rat Terrier puppy. Living on a small farm may sound like a dream, but our land was for pigs and cattle. One thing farmers did not buy was a puppy. For starters, they cost way too much.

The puppy I found was in the classified ads in the Sunday paper that I scoured every week after church while the football game was on. There they were: Rat Terrier puppies in Redwood Falls, Minnesota, only a five-hour drive away. And one more thing: They cost $150. This was in 1980 and any money for a puppy was too much according to my father, but my mother (who never really liked dogs but did love me) persuaded him to get the puppy because she was very worried about my well-being.

One of my earlier dogs that I loved dearly was a Rat Terrier named Freckles. From the start, I was deeply connected with that dog. On a warm summer's day, I saw Freckles playing in the field across the road, most likely chasing mice or chipmunks. I called her across the dirt road. I didn't see a car fast approaching until it was too late and Freckles was hit. I will never forget the sound, the site, or my scream to alert her. Anything to save her precious life.

I held her in a blanket the entire way to town as my dad drove her to see Dr. Stenzland, our veterinarian. I was told he could not save her, but he could give her a shot to relieve her pain and allow her to pass peacefully.

It was too much to bear, too much to see, too much think about and *there was absolutely no trying. No one tried to save her.* Even the news of that was just too much. An operation was too much money, and there was not enough hope to take that financial risk.

Freckles died because I called her across the road and *no one tried to save her.* The pain was unbearable.

I buried her under our trees out behind our farm buildings. Afterwards, I would visit her daily at her grave until I graduated and moved away to college. I still miss her and sob when I think of her. So much more could have been done. *No one even tried.*

That is why a new puppy was so important to my mother who insisted I adopt a new friend because it would (maybe) get me to stop thinking about Freckles. Maybe I would stop sitting by her grave. Maybe I would be able to sleep again at night.

We drove to Redwood Falls and picked up Samantha. Three days later, Sam, became very ill with parvovirus, a life-threatening virus that can kill dogs, especially puppies. I was only 12 and demanded that my parents pay the vet.

"You're not letting my dog die," I cried.

Where there's a will …

Dr. Stenzland examined Sam and he placed her on IV fluids and kept her for five days. My father paid him to save my Sam and this time Dr. Stenzland did. She rebounded and lived a long, healthy life.

Again, when someone tells me, "You have no idea how much my pet means to me," I do, I really do. I feel that statement in my heart, in my soul and it resonates and makes me choke on my words because that is the very reason I became a veterinarian. I want to make sure that every patient; every child and every person who loves an animal has a chance. I wanted to make sure the face they saw working on their beloved animal cared as much as they did.

That is what everyone deserves.

Someone who cares as much as they do.

It wasn't too long before I was 21 and holding a fresh degree in biology and philosophy in hand from Hamline University in St. Paul, Minnesota. After college, I took some time to work as a naturalist and volunteered helping others hike the wilds of Northern Minnesota. I lived in a cabin and people would come, stay and hike into the Boundary Waters Canoe Area. I'm not sure why I took this position, except that I can be a granola girl at times. There were a lot of black bears and moose around and I'm happy to report I never ran into any of them or treated them. We just happily co-existed!

Back in civilization, I worked for a vaccine development company in research before deciding to pursue my Masters at The University of Southern Mississippi and then on to my Doctorate in Veterinary Medicine at the University of Minnesota.

As a young veterinarian in training, my heart was with my patients. In fact, I found out how vulnerable you can be when your body (human or animal) isn't cooperating. During my final year of veterinary school, I went in for a routine pap smear that came back with bad news. It was cancerous. I had a biopsy and I was told, "You may need to have a hysterectomy." I always longed to be a mother and prayed this wasn't the case. In the end, the doctors didn't need to take my entire uterus out, but instead removed only part of my cervix. I was told that I could still have children, which was a relief.

Two days after the procedure was done, I was in my gratitude mode at an animal hospital *externing* (sort of like interning), which is what one does during their last year of vet school. I went to open a cage door where a docile (at least it looked that way) Cocker Spaniel was resting inside. For no real reason, the dog lunged and in a nanosecond bit me so hard that her teeth sunk through my thumb joint. In blinding pain, I was rushed to the emergency room.

That night, I was on my antibiotics, hand bandaged and back at the large animal veterinary teaching hospital where I had the evening shift, which meant you were there for emergencies and to check on the animals who were staying overnight. At one in the morning, I was working with another vet student named Doug and we were refluxing a horse.

A quick anatomy lesson: Thanks to their unique bodies, horses cannot vomit, so when they have fluid build-up in their stomachs, a veterinarian must place a tube down their nose and throat to the stomach to get the fluid out. So, there I was holding onto this horse that didn't want a tube down his nose when Doug says, "Melissa, what are those red lines running up and down your arm?"

"Oh my gosh," I said, gazing at them. I was so busy with the horse that I didn't have time to deal with the fact that my arm felt vaguely warmer than usual. "I'm septic. I have a blood infection from the bite," I said in a matter-of-fact voice.

We finished with the horse and I calmly said, "Doug, I hate to leave you alone here, but I have to go to the hospital now – the people hospital. Good night."

I was admitted despite the fact that I smelled like a barn. A few X-rays later I was on an IV and a hand surgeon was called. "This wound needs to be flushed out," the doctor told me, 'Or you could lose your thumb." Calmly, I explained that I was finishing vet school and needed all of my fingers to do surgery.

The hand surgeon specialist, a beautiful man out of a GQ photo spread, walked in, examined my hand and sniffed hard. I could see the poor man's eyes watering. "I'm sorry," he finally said to me. "But what is that smell?"

"It's horse," I said.

"Horse?" he questioned.

"I was refluxing a horse…before I came in…after I was bit by a Cocker Spaniel…It's been a very long and exciting day," I said.

I said it like this was the most normal 24-hour span in the world.

To me, it was.

After four days in the hospital, I was sprung into my uncertain future, but thankfully with a healing thumb. My life was at a crossroads when I was offered an internship in California. I didn't know what to do. I turned that offer down. Life intervened and I found another internship in Boston. A few weeks later, my thumb was working just fine (whew) and I was moving to Bean Town, one of America's great cities.

Life for a young veterinarian is grueling because on these necessary internships you're paid less than minimum wage or about $263 a week. I was given a room to live in, which in my case was the upstairs of the veterinary hospital. I had a wonderful roommate who owned two rats and I moved in with two beloved friends, my Basenjis, Toby and Cleo. They were my buds and got me through everything in life. My rocks.

I worked at a very busy hospital, just outside of the city, where it wasn't unusual for me to put in 120 hours a week including many overnight shifts. Most of my days were about 12 to 18 hours long depending on what emergency walked in or was carried in. It was a lot, but I reminded myself that human beings could do anything for one year.

The experience was amazing and I learned quickly that pets and people are intricately connected. I was young and looked young, so many clients thought I was "too young" to help their beloved pet. The trust had to be built and built quickly, otherwise the client wouldn't allow me to do anything. Rightly so, these pets meant the world to them.

I learned how to show I cared deeply because I did.

One night, a gentleman came in on emergency because his Golden Retriever was covered in bugs. This sounded terrible, so I quickly went into the exam room to examine Daisy. Daisy was a beautiful Golden with fluffy, well-groomed fur of a deep blonde color and a very happy face. I could see her smile when I entered the room. She didn't fuss when I examined her from head to tail. I couldn't find bugs. I couldn't find anything; she was in perfect condition.

I explored more with the client and he insisted she was covered in bugs and couldn't believe I could not see them. Instead of getting frustrated, I asked him to point out one of the bugs on Daisy. My client tried and tried again, but he couldn't find any bugs. Then, he broke down and started to cry. He picked up his phone and dialed a number and asked me to speak with his daughter.

"Hello, this is Dr. Magnuson and I have Daisy and your dad here and he is very concerned that Daisy is covered in bugs, but I cannot find any bugs on Daisy," I said.

The daughter then asked me "Is Daisy okay? Is my father ok?"

"Yes, they both appear perfectly fine, but your father seems very sad."

The daughter's voice became shaky and quiet.

"My father is dying of bone cancer and he is on liquid morphine because the pain is so bad," she said. "It makes him hallucinate. I am very sorry he has wasted your time. I will come pick both of them up."

I sat in silence.

Not sure what to say.

"Thank you for telling me, I will make sure Daisy and your father wait here until you arrive," I said.

Then, I hung up the phone.

I had a long heart-felt conversation with Daisy's father. He explained to me what it was like to be dying, how scared he was and how Daisy gave him a reason to live and get up each day.

"Daisy doesn't judge," he said. "She just loves me and understands right where I am…each step of the way.

"I'll miss her when I'm gone – and my family," he said. "But I know the time is coming to say good-bye."

Daisy just sat by the man's side, licking his hand. She put her head on his knee. Smiled up at him.

Daisy and Dad were connected.

I understood.

What got me through my internship, perpetual learning and working 120 hours per week was the love of Toby and Cleo. On my off hours, I'd walk them everywhere. I'd say hello to people who looked at me like I was crazy. I guess this wasn't the norm on the East Coast, but I'm a Midwesterner by heart. Around the hospital, the reception was far better because for the first time, I was being called the name I dreamt of as a kid.

"Hello, Dr. Magnuson," I'd hear.

Even early in my career, I began to describe myself as a Conscious Vet – someone who really cares about what is happening with animals and animal medicine and who is proactive about furthering advancement in health care for all creatures great and small. At each of my three hospitals now, we are there to treat the whole family. It's not necessarily just about the pet. It's also about the owner and how much information they can give me as the voice of their animal companion.

You speak for them. I try to connect the pieces of the puzzle that you give me.

I try to heal them.

It's a good team.

After my grueling year as an intern, I wasn't certain I wanted to take a full-time position just yet. Yet, I loved emergency medicine, surgery, exotic animals and working with the clients. I interviewed at several hospitals, but did not feel any were the right fit for me. That's why I spent a year doing relief work (working for veterinarians when they were on vacation), so I could get a feel for many hospitals. Quickly, I learned I did not want to work for anyone else. I enjoyed being my own boss, setting my own hours, and above all, I wanted to practice a high standard of veterinary medicine and prove to the client that I truly cared.

In 2000, I opened my house-call practice. This was an adventure. Not only was I seeing pets in their own home setting, but also, I was seeing the client and observing how everyone lived.

One of my elderly clients, Ms. Anna, had a hip replacement and was in a wheelchair and recovering. She lived in a very old, lovely Cape house with perfect white shutters and a cottage garden.

Ms. Anna owned Felicity, a feral cat. A feral cat is a cat that has been captured or trapped from outdoor living, spayed or neutered, given its vaccines and is typically returned to the outdoors. Felicity, who was believed to be "a bit friendlier," was placed in a residential home.

Ms. Anna adopted this cat from a local cat rescue. The rescue thought Ms. Anna's home would be perfect because it was very quiet and small, plus the attention of an elderly woman who was home all the time could be good for the cat. When I arrived at Ms. Anna's house with my technician, we soon noticed that all the doors on the interior of the house had been removed because of Ms. Anna's wheelchair. This was a very old house with narrow doorways and in order for Ms. Anna to navigate in and out of rooms, the doors had to be removed. Even the bathroom door was gone.

Now, anyone who has ever tried to catch a cat before knows that you typically try to place the cat in one small room in order to quickly scoop up the animal for an exam. This house had no doors, which meant no rooms to corral a cat, especially not a feral cat that was used to survival skills and running from anything she thought may be a predator.

While my technician and I tried to corner the cat in any small room, Felicity was much smarter than two humans. She would dart over, under, around and through making her capture almost impossible.

"Ms. Anna, it's going to be very hard for me to capture Felicity without any doors. Will she come to you?" I asked.

This frail woman who was daintily dressed said, "Oh no, Felicity beats to her own drummer. I've had her for three years and I have never even touched her! We just talk."

Silence…again.

Not sure of my response.

"The town says I have to get her rabies vaccinated or they will come take her," Ms. Anna fretted. "But she is so lovely and she is my best friend. So, I need her to have that vaccine."

"You must catch her," she instructed.

She was her best friend. They talk. She lives alone.

There was no choice. I would catch the feral cat in the house with no doors.

My technician and I spent an hour trying to outsmart a six-pound feline. Somehow, by sheer stroke of luck, we were finally able to trap her in the bathtub and wrapped her in Ms. Anna's beautiful, luxury Houndstooth blanket. Felicity wasn't happy, while Ms. Anna was overjoyed. I did a very quick check-up followed by the rabies vaccine and Felicity was "legal" to stay in Ms. Anna's home.

Ms. Anna passed away several years later and prior to her death, she asked me to place Felicity in a proper home where I thought she would do well. Ms. Anna's daughter delivered the cat to me (I have no idea how she caught her!) and she lived at my vet hospital for two weeks. During this time, Felicity escaped her kennel enclosure twice, set the alarms off in the middle of night and caused the police to case the place for intruders…only to find Felicity darting over, under, around and through the police officers.

This made me smile on the inside.

I did find Felicity a proper home with an elderly gentleman who lost his cat several months earlier. Mr. George immediately fell in love with Felicity and was even able to pet her.

It was a happy ending for all.

I opened my first veterinary hospital five years after starting my house-call practice. House calls were filled up and the only way I could accommodate more clients was to have a building where people could bring their pets to see me. I purchased a small piece of land with a little house that I renovated into a homey veterinary practice.

I closed on the property from my hospital bed, September 28, 2005, the same day I gave birth to my third daughter. Just a few months later that December, I opened Canobie Lake Veterinary Hospital.

My three daughters grew up in my hospital. I had a room upstairs completely outfitted as a toy room and my nanny watched them while I saw appointments and did surgery. I was lucky to be able to pop in and out to see them during the day.

One of my other colleagues, who also owned her veterinary practice, would share stories of pets, people and our children. Dr. Miller, a great vet and friend, called me one day to get advice.

"I just got off the phone with Timmy's teacher," she said as we discussed her six-year-old son. "She wants to have a face-to-face meeting with me."

She went on to explain, "The teacher asked the children today what happens to pets when they die and Timmy raised his hand and said 'I know, I know! They go in my mom's freezer.'"

I burst out laughing, but I did feel Dr. Miller's pain. The teacher could only imagine what Dr. Miller was doing with animals in her freezer! Veterinarian's children know that when pets die, they smell so they are stored in the hospital freezer specifically for this reason until the cremation service picks them up. Little Timmy thought he was sharing really good information and assumed everyone's mom did this on a daily basis.

Four years after opening my first hospital, a local shelter asked me to open a hospital in their rental space. I had been volunteering my time at the shelter for several years.

In June of 2009, I opened All Pets Veterinary Hospital. It wasn't long before I had outgrown this rental space and moved All Pets to a 5000-square foot dream hospital with state of the art equipment and facilities. After the move from the small shelter space to the new beautiful building, one of my All Pets clients told me, "Now, your building matches your level of care."

What a compliment because the building was absolutely stunning.

In 2012, a friend of mine asked me to purchase an animal hospital because the veterinarian was retiring. This was an adorable vet hospital on the Seacoast of New Hampshire and had a very similar footprint to my Canobie Hospital. It was homey and had a wonderful hometown clientele. In May of that year, I purchased Greenland Veterinary Hospital.

My plate was full.

Many ask me, "How do you do all you do?" I do all I do because I am surrounded by amazing staff, friends, and clients. My clients (and patients) have taught me so much about medicine and life. They help me manage it all.

Having three hospitals means that I have a lot of interesting stories about the amazing world of animals.

Belgarian was a large, very large, fluffy and formidable Alaskan Malamute weighing in at 150 pounds. His owners were a lovely couple in the military. They owned two of these large breed dogs, plus four cats. Now, everyone in the veterinary world knows that Malamutes and cats should never be in the same home together. Malamutes have a very strong prey drive and often will kill cats.

Not in this house.

Belgarian and his fellow Malamute buddy knew their distinct roles in this family and also knew how important those kitty cats were to mom in this house. How did they know? Dad told them and told them frequently. Dad was a confident man with a calm demeanor and a heart bigger than Belgarian. When Dad spoke, everyone listened.

During one of my house-calls at their house, "BW" -- black and white cat-- was not feeling well. I examined BW and needed to draw blood and get a urine sample. BW did not like being held by a technician, so he was resisting restraint and wanted to get away. BW let out a yowl and Belgarian came bounding at me to rescue BW, his kitty. Dad, the calm military captain yelled from his gut at

Belgarian, "SIT DOWN!".

I sat down.

Then I realized, so did Belgarian. There I was sitting trying to decide if I was more scared of Belgarian or Dad?

We all sat in silence. Even BW was quiet. I stood up, drew the blood and completed my tasks. Belgarian stayed put. He listened to his leader and respected his command.

All of the animals in this house understood their unique roles and their connections with both mom and dad. These were some of the most loved and cared for pets I have ever vetted. This house exuded love and a caring aura. You felt it the moment you walked in.

This was how I wanted my veterinary hospitals to be. From the moment you walk in, I want you to know we care and understand the special connection each and every person has with his or her pet; and that it means something different to each person. In turn, I promise there will be love and kindness with each pet we have in our care.

Of course, so many times the pets are the ones doing the most of the caring and teaching.

I learn a lot from animals.

You might be wondering exactly who lives with me besides my amazing husband Andy and wonderful children, Emma, Elise and Eva – ages from 12 to 16. Here's the list of my other "kids":

Boo – Mini Australian Shepherd
Lola – Chihuahua
Luigi – Italian Greyhound
Stella – Mini Australian Shepherd
Kiwi – Tortoise Shell Cat
Henry – Meyers Parrot

King Tut – Guinea Pig

Rio –Bearded Dragon

And a partridge in a pear tree – just kidding!

Zoobiquity

Animals and people have such an astonishing connection that a term was created to describe it called zoobiquity. Coined by human cardiologist Barbara Natterson-Horowitz and medical author Kathryn Bowers, the word describes a species-spanning approach to health that draws expertise from veterinary and human medicine.

My take on zoobiquity boils it down to the scientific fact that we, as humans, not only experience some of the same medical issues as our animals, but we also share quite similar emotions and understandings of life. We have a lot to learn from our animal counterparts.

To put it simply: Animal and human life often run on parallel courses. We need to intersect these lives more often because of the wealth of knowledge it will bring.

As a veterinarian, I find this beyond fascinating and it informs my practice each and every day. At the core, I figure it this way: Yes, I'm saving pet lives, but in turn I'm saving pet people because the connection between those on two legs and four paws is that strong and unbreakable.

This connection is also difficult to define.

Scientists have studied animals with the help of ingenious experiments to explore the mental capabilities of hundreds of species. One famous study was that of Irene Pepperberg and her African grey parrot, Alex.

Alex lived to be 31 and learned more than 100 words while he also differentiated between shapes and colors. Scientists were reticent to accept that Alex was "intelligent," but it certainly sparked interest in the area that animals were actually quite smart and warranted looking into further.

Prior to Pepperberg's work, Jane Goodall, with much resistance from the scientific community, showed how chimpanzees had thoughtful and emotional lives and brought to the forefront our animal connections in many ways. These included everything from rich personalities to complex social relationships.

I would argue that our pets, whether we believe they are intelligent, smart, emotional or thoughtful, or whatever word you choose, are actually "connected." The connection that Dr. Pepperberg had with Alex and Dr. Goodall with many chimpanzees produced oodles of research and inferences into animal behavior, intelligence, perception, and I would add consciousness or the ability to be self-aware.

Self-awareness is the capacity to recognize oneself as an individual separate from the environment and others. Scientists in the past have believed that "The Mirror Test" was the way to determine self-recognition. If an animal can use a mirror to find body parts otherwise hidden from sight, they are thought to recognize themselves in a mirror and thus are "self-aware." Many animals like gorillas, orangutans, elephants, dolphins, magpies, and manta rays have passed the mirror test. This self-recognition has been tested in many species, even fish, and they have found that smell is used to recognize themselves and others because their habitat in which they live is a low visibility water world and visual cues are a less valued sense.

Many scientists now believe that self-awareness may be a capacity that all vertebrates and even insects possess. I would argue that this self-awareness is something animals can teach us, not us teaching them.

Just like Dr. Natterson-Horowitz and Kathryn Bowers believe animal and human commonality can be used to diagnose, treat, and heal patients of all species, I believe we can even go further and say that our pets are actually teaching us to be more animal-like; we need to look at our animal nature (animality) and explore this connectedness. This connection will actually help or perhaps catapult humans into true consciousness.

A DEEPER CONNECTION

Our species are connected in so many ways. Quite often, we share similar diseases, emotional ticks and, yes, you can even start looking like your pet – or vice versa. I would call your relationship with your animal a spiritual one, too. Think about it: Quite often your pet can become one of the closest living creatures in your world. Your pet or animal companion can have the most profound effect on your daily life. We wake up with our pets, eat with them, work beside them quite often, relax with them, play with them and then call it a night with them…only to place this whole thing on repeat the next day.

As our relationship with our animal merges into a gelled living experience together, you will find your pet even mimicking your emotions, diseases, ups, downs, joys and heartbreaks. You're sad; they're sad, you're jumping up and down, so are they – but more on that in future chapters.

If you're going to have this type of close relationship with any living thing, it's helpful to start at the very beginning. Why that dog? Why that cat…or lizard or rabbit? How did this human, and that animal find each other in the first place and make the leap to form a family? What was the first link of this unique, lifelong bond?

Choosing what animal comes into your realm is one of life's major decisions because what you're really doing is marrying your personality to that of your pet. I'm not saying to rush out and find an animal that is exactly like you. In fact, your pet might be quite opposite of you in many areas, but at the same time will be the perfect learning experience or right fit.

You might read this and think, "Nah, Dr. Melissa. I've always been a Labrador Retriever type of person." Or I hear, "I can't live without a 20-pound white Poodle." Again, it goes back to linking your inner self with what's special about those animals that compliment you emotionally. In many ways, the relationship with your pet mirrors how you pick your love mate in human form. Maybe you're exactly like your husband or your wife is the direct opposite of you. But in the end, it works. It actually feels perfect and meant to be.

The same goes with the creatures in your life and the lives of your family members.

DO WE REALLY CHOOSE OUR ANIMAL COMPANIONS?

In a word, no.

I don't believe we actually choose a pet like we scoop up those three extra red apples in the produce aisle and then move onto the next task in life. With the apples, you're looking for perfection – ripe, red, firm. Animals don't come with those kinds of labels. I think we are drawn to certain animals for reasons that only a specific individual can understand. It comes down to a feeling or an instinct that this is "the one."

As a vet, I can often pinpoint (without even asking) the exact reason why someone had an urge to adopt that specific animal while leaving those other adorable dogs and cats for someone else to adopt.

Sometimes, what matches physically and feels familiar may be the reason. For instance, I have a client who has four small white dogs of different breeds, but they all look exactly the same. It's no coincidence that she is a small, white haired older lady. In many ways, they look like the perfect pack with the human as the alpha. All four of her little dogs show a specific part of her personality. One is very well dressed with her fancy groomed hair coat (this woman dresses well); one is very confident in his actions (she is a very well-grounded individual); the third dog is aloof to most of the world around her (this woman is very calm and centered in most situations); and her last dog has a host of medical issues which is why she sees me (mirroring her husband whom she also cares for around the clock.)

Then there is a male client of mine who is a sandy haired, medium sized, middle-aged man with three buff colored dogs – a Cocker, a Golden Doodle and a dusty colored Poodle. It's almost as if they're all wearing the same coat! The tough guy down the block walks his tough looking German Shepherd. Deep down, the guy and the dog are two big softies who like to hunker down on the couch together and sneak late-night snacks. It's another case of like attracting like.

In other cases, you might see that stick-thin young woman walking that huge Great Dane. Maybe they don't look alike, but the fact that they're both gentle beings figures into it. That restless athlete runs every morning with his Border Collie because they both have energy to burn and hate being cooped up. The bonds were there from moment one.

Let's say you're ready to invite a new animal into your life. You've made the decision that this is a true bond and that you will be there for that animal for its entire life and care for it properly while treating it like a family member.

The question remains: How do you pick the perfect pet?

Answer: You don't. They pick you.

ANIMALS ARE KNOWING

It doesn't matter if you're standing in front of a shelter cage gazing at those fully-grown beauties or at a breeder's kennels looking at that adorable new litter of cats or dogs. Of course, there are so many choices – some adorable and others heartbreaking. It might seem overwhelming because many of us have a natural instinct to want to adopt them all. But, that's not really possible. And choosing the right animal companion isn't really that mind boggling, if you take a breath and let it just happen.

You might start by asking a few questions: What dogs come up to you? Which ones back away? Maybe there is one who even growls? What cat curls around your legs? Which one runs for the hills? Which one just nags at you because it feels so right?

Choosing your new pet shouldn't be a rushed type of endeavor. You didn't just drive the car to a certain spot, look at a row of women or men and pick a life mate in the time it takes to order a fresh Starbucks. This pet is about to become a big part of your household, someone you will spend hours with each day over several years, so allow the time to let the situation unfold.

Yes, that breeder might insist that there are only two puppies left or a certain type of cat is rare in your town, so you should take him or her. Don't let anyone rush you into a snap decision. Take a minute. Take a deep breath. Take a few deep breaths. And enjoy spending a little time with animals, which is one of life's joys. Sit down on the floor with groups of them. Claim your spot in the grass. Let them come to you.

Think of this as a story that's on page one, but don't flip to the next chapter too quickly. Some animals are shy and need a moment to smell you and make sure you're okay and harmless. How sad to miss out on that one great dog, who just needs a few minutes to come out of his or her shell. Maybe you're shy, too. It's not always the most outgoing animal that's the fit. This is about a mesh of many things including personalities and intentions.

Resolve that you might not find that perfect pet today, but tomorrow they will be waiting. I tell many clients who are looking for their next pet to just put it out there into the universe and you will be amazed at how that pet will find you.

I have a client who spent several months going to different breeders in the Chicago suburbs to look at female German Shepherds. She saw a lot of cute dogs that she could have easily scooped up, but deep in her heart she never met *her* dog. Even her husband was exasperated and said, "I want a dog in the house. These are gorgeous puppies. Let me choose." But she stood firm, insisting that one day she would *just know* when the dog was right. Five months into their search, there was a lone female pup in a litter of all males born to a local doctor. Her face was a bit scratched up from playing roughly with her brothers, but my client knew that it was meant to be. Cody lived to be 17-years-old and was, in her words, "the best dog in the world. A true soulmate. I can't imagine how life would have been for either of us if I would have made a snap decision on my first one or two stops and adopted another dog."

I can't stress enough how important it is that you feel a connection when choosing a pet. Feel it in your heart and bones. This is your "instinct" working with your new pet's "instinct." You know when you know. You just know in the moment that this is your pet. So many clients have asked me why this happens and I believe the reason is simple: You feel that tug or pull towards that animal because the animal is actually choosing you. Take your longing for an animal and their instincts and it equals a connection that's unique for every person… and for every animal that has chosen their human companion.

Personally, I love how these connections work themselves out, even when it seems that they will not.

Gale is a wonderful woman who runs one of my hospitals and breeds Mini Australian Shepherds. I had a client whose Aussie died and she asked me to recommend a responsible breeder in the area. Immediately, I told her about Gale and quickly my client was on the line asking if she had any tri-colored pups.

"I only have a red one left," Gale said.

My client wasn't sure, but she had a feeling that she should meet the red one although her heart was set on a tri-color.

"Can we come look?" she asked.

Wouldn't you know it, but exactly one tri-color was still there waiting for a new owner to pick her up. My client spent some time playing with her and fell in love. The feeling was mutual, but the tri was spoken for already. Even when my client went to leave, that knowing little tri was attempting to follow her out of a big door in order to "go home." At the same time, the little red female was cute, but it wasn't the same sort of connection, so my client went home to think about the red one knowing it wasn't really her dog. The next day, she decided to adopt it anyways. During that time, the people who adopted the tri-colored one, picked her up. A few days later, Gale's phone rang because these new owners had "an issue."

The husband, it turns out, felt a deeper bond with the red pup.

"I love the little red dog," he said. "Is there any way….."

Fate conspired and both couples found themselves at the breeders again. Gale quickly gave the red dog to the first couple and they were thrilled. My client couldn't believe that the tri-colored one was now available and scooped her up within seconds. They literally swapped dogs – and lived happily ever after with the pets that were meant for each family.

I heard the story and just smiled, but I wasn't surprised. I just put it in the mental file I call Miraculous Ways Animals Make Their Way Into The Right Human Lives.

THE DOOR OPENS

Pets come into our lives in mysterious ways. It had been a very busy day at my hospital where we had several "drop off" appointments meaning working clients will drop off their pet for treatment or an exam during the day. One such day, a caregiver had dropped off Harold because his owner had passed away.

Harold was a 12-year old cat with dirty white and black fur. He curled himself up in the corner of the cage with his head tucked into his legs and slept. He was very thin and when I felt his abdomen, I could feel his colon was very distended with poop.

"Where is the paperwork for Harold?" I asked my staff. "Is it euthanasia paperwork?"

"His owner died and there is no one to care for him," my technician explained.

I looked at Harold and he looked at me. It certainly did seem like he didn't feel well, but it didn't seem like it was time for him to pass.

Another technician named Heidi looked at Harold and chimed in.

"He looks perfectly fine. We can't euthanize him?" she said.

Here was the dilemma: An owner signed off to have their pet euthanized, but I didn't see a medical reason to do it. Yes, hair coat was a little rough, plus he seemed very dehydrated and constipated, but these were not reasons to put Harold to sleep.

Heidi immediately said, "I will take him, I will call the caregiver."

Heidi made that call and found that the caregiver was very excited to find out that someone wanted Harold and was willing to care for him. In a split second, Heidi and Harold became best friends and she cared for him for four more years. He immediately became a pack member of her family and within months was no longer thin and had a beautiful hair coat.

I asked Heidi the big question.

"How did you decide so quickly that you wanted to take Harold home?"

"I didn't decide," she said. "One look and Harold decided for me."

Later, I asked her what Harold taught her while he was in her care.

"We are not our pets' masters," she said. "I learned that we are just privileged to be part of their world."

What brings people and that specific pet together?

Maybe it's that lost dog that you found. Or perhaps it's your neighbor who can no longer keep her cat and gives you the best pet of your entire life. Maybe it's a force that's greater than any of us. Your job as the human is to just source out the signs. Listen to your intuition because, again, your relationship with your animal is based on a much higher connection than just emotions. If a certain animal is pretty and nice, but you don't feel it…then don't do it.

That animal belongs with someone else.

Keep an eye out for animals that approach you as it's important to recognize an animal that is trying to enter your life. It's that dog that keeps showing up on your front lawn and then you find out the owners don't really want it anymore. It's that call you get from a distant relation saying, "I don't know why I thought of you, but I think you need to see these puppies." You go visit and that one puppy is standoffish, but then slowly inches his way up and then jumps into your lap. That pet with the hopeful face and wagging tail is offering you everything – body, heart, soul – and their very lives.

HOW DO THEY PICK YOU?

How does that pet know you're *that* person? They just do. It's amazing, but most animals just have that intuitive connection that indicates that this feels right or wrong. Call it a sixth sense. They listen to it more than we listen to it. As humans, we can have "a feeling" and often choose to either ignore it or act on it later or never.

Animals live in *the now*. If they have a feeling or instinct, they're jumping on it – right in that moment. They also don't judge. They don't care if you're rich or poor, fat or thin or live in the best part of town or the worst. They're about unconditional love, which can live anywhere as long as you live there.

There is a very important lesson for people to learn, which is pets find us with no judgement. As a veterinary professional, we need to remember not to judge a person's animal connection. About a year ago, I was walking the streets of Manhattan with my family on a New York vacation. There was a man in a wheelchair with tattered clothing, holes in his shoes and he smelled as if he may not have showered for weeks. He had three small Chihuahuas and a grey and white cat that sat in his lap as he slowly tiptoed his wheelchair down the streets. He was old, disheveled and dirty but his eyes and smile lit up the street.

None of the animals were leashed, yet all of them stayed by his side. Each of them would periodically jump down, run around his wheelchair and jump back up. This even included the cat! Two of the Chihuahuas would run back and forth at one another and antagonize the cat. The cat would jump down and swipe at the large Chihuahua and he would give out a yip. Then they would all jump back up into the man's lap and cuddle.

I watched intently for a long time. This family of five needed each other, loved each other, and found each other...all connected and exuded a beautiful loving relationship. Many would judge this, but in its purest form, this group was meant to be together.

HOW THEY "TALK"

Since pets can't speak, they quite often grab us with their paws or rub against us during that first meeting while other animals in the room just ignore us. One client was looking at new feline friends. One kept winding in and out of her legs; the other kept jumping into a nearby trash can.

In many cases that insistent pet is saying to you, "Okay, you're mine. Don't you feel it? Come on! We've got this thing together. Take me home."

If that same pet could just wander into your home they would ……..and they would make it their own. They feel something in your energy, some call it unconditional love, and it matches their own vibe.

This is why I'm not a fan of breeders picking out your pet because of color or sex. You can't order a dog or cat like you're ordering a pizza. It can't be: "I'll take a cute brown one with three white spots and all her shots." Finding the right new family member runs so much deeper than allowing a third party to pick for you. This could result in a big mistake or missing out on an important life relationship.

I always think this beginning part is meant to be – or not meant to be, which is why we pass on other pets. Glenn, a 60-year-old widower, lost his beloved Baxter, a 13-year-old Shepherd mix. He went to the local pound again and again, feeling guilty each time for not picking a new companion.

"I just didn't feel it, although there were so many dogs that needed a loving home," he said. A few weeks later, a local rescue group he works with introduced him to Ava, a six-month Lab pup, who had an unfavorable beginning. There was this feeling he had when this shy girl took the chance to lick his hand. Immediately, he adopted her, nursed her back to health and the two are inseparable.

"When it's right, you just know it," he said. "She will never replace Baxter in my heart, but this is an entirely different and just as important journey that's meant to be for both of us."

I like to tell clients that one pet will never replace or have the same place in your heart as another pet. They will, however, find a new spot in your heart that needs filling.

At the hospital, we had an owner come in with a red, 10-year-old Burmese cat, which are quite rare. A few months prior, she had a new baby and the cat was terrified each time the baby cried. The cat was so upset with the crying that it was getting sick and even stopped eating. The owner was heartbroken, but knew that her cat wouldn't make it if this continued. I kept the cat at the hospital to nurse it back to health and put a notice on Facebook that it was up for adoption to a home that could handle her medical care.

A few days later, I got a phone call from a woman in Colorado who was desperate to find a red Burmese. I gave her just a bit of information, but she cut right to the chase. "This is my cat. I just know it," she told me with such sureness in her voice that I even knew it was absolutely right. "What should I do? I'll send you money," she begged. "I'll get on a plane and come and get my cat. I just need two days. Please don't allow anyone else to adopt her. We would both be missing out."

I didn't even want money and neither did the original owner. If this woman cared enough to buy a plane ticket, I was fairly certain this cat was going to have a lovely life. I encouraged her to come and get her new pet. Deep down, I hoped that she was serious and, most importantly, felt a connection when she held the cat for the first time.

Two days later, she was in my waiting room with an excited smile on her face. The cat was let loose, actually ran immediately to this stranger and cuddled right into her neck. It's years later and the woman still sends me pictures of her and the Burmese sharing their happy lives together, which was a sweet ending for one family and a new beginning for another.

Moral of the story: Pets have a way of finding us. This is despite the odds including distance, financial concerns or other particulars. This is why when clients need to re-home their pet for whatever reason, I understand. It just means the pet has done their job where they are and are meant to have a connection with someone else.

I can't tell you how many times I've been told this story: "I held about 20 dogs, one more adorable than the next, but this one melted into my arms and then wrapped her front legs around me like a hug." Or, "I looked at dozens of cats, but this one looked up at me and I just knew that we had this link. It was meant to be for both of us."

Think of it like the animal world's version of a sped up Match.com. When an animal knows, they're going to act on it and fast. If that dog or cat isn't a hugger or snuggle type, they might show it by a look on their face, a purr, a sigh or by simply coming back to you again and again while almost pushing the other furry creatures out of the way. When an animal finds you, they want to close the deal and start their life with you together.

Your pet finds you, they are there to teach you valuable lessons, most of which, you don't even know you need to learn or are going to happen. These lessons are different for everyone in the household. Animals have a beautiful way of "reading you" and understanding you. This is why your pet connection is so strong. They see the connection and teach you how it is to be built. We simply need to listen.

Remember that most animals are territorial. When they stake a claim, they're going to keep coming back until the deal is done. But for the animal, it's done when they feel it. They've chosen. You're "It."

One note: I'm a big believer that the adults in the family should ultimately choose the pet. It's tougher to decide by committee. But if you are looking at pets for a specific family member or child, pay close attention to the interactions with different members of the family. There is not always a spiritual connection with everyone in the pack and that's fine in these cases because you're selecting that cat for your daughter or son.

Sometimes there is no connection with Mom and Dad, but that's okay because that pet's main person feels it. If you're adopting a pet for the entire family then start by letting one of the adults feel the bond and make the decision. Animals connect differently with every member of the family. A pet's purpose is different for each member of the family. Perhaps Fifi never licks your face, but she always licks your daughter's face. That's because Fifi has a different connection or purpose with each family member.

At our home, my Chihuahua was adopted for my oldest daughter who immediately bonded with this dog. There was no choice, but this animal for her. Sure, she's warm and friendly with the rest of the family, but the dog would like nothing better than to be one step ahead or behind my daughter the entire day, 365 days a year. In the same way, our red Aussie prefers to be with either my youngest child or me.

I have this wonderful couple, two men, who are very, very, very meticulous about their appearances. When I met them, it looked like they could go right from my vet hospital to the swankiest restaurant in town or a photo shoot. (I've never been to their home, but I imagine it's something out of Architectural

Digest.) You can imagine how it shocked me when they brought in a new pet, a cat, that was an unruly mess. The poor kitty was dirty with matted hair.

"My grandmother died and there was no one to take care of her beloved cat. She begged us to keep it, plus the cat would never leave us alone when we visited during her last days. The cat was practically in our arms demanding to go with us," Gary told me.

"We're not pet people," cautioned his partner Bob. "But it breaks my heart even thinking of taking her beloved cat to a shelter. Can you help us because we've never had a cat or any other pet?" Since the grandmother was sick, the cat was undernourished and her fur was a dull, tangled mess. The good news was there were no other major health issues and we were able to easily fix the cosmetic issues with a good grooming.

My clients did everything I asked to bring this kitty back to her full splendor including dietary changes and grooming techniques. A year later, they came in with their little "baby" who fit neatly into Gary's well-dressed arms.

I wasn't shocked.

The cat looked like it could be in a TV commercial. It was perfect. Pristine. The fur almost gleamed because it was so shiny and silky. Her weight was ideal. Her eyes were bright and shiny. On second glance, I looked at my clients and then the cat again. They could *all* show up at a palace and no one would have blinked an eye. "We love our cat," Bob told me. "She's like our child now."

It was beyond obvious that this clever feline picked them for this part of her life – and life was very good for all involved.

They said they weren't "pet people."

That cat knew the truth. They were her people.

Let's go back to zoobiquity or how we're all connected in ways we might not even realize at first. There are cases of new pet relationships that occur and connect within the same house with principals who have been in each other's living space forever.

In my practice, I spent years doing check-ups on a lizard that belonged to a young boy. The only thing is little boys who love their animal companions grow up and go to college and lizards are not allowed in most dorm rooms. Heartbroken, this young man begged his mother – a non-reptile person as she always insisted – to take care of his beloved Molly the lizard in his absence. He promised that, of course, he would take over during winter and summer vacations. Mom was sad because she was not only letting her son go, but was also "stuck" – as she told me on her first solo visit to the vet—taking care of this scale-y thing.

A funny thing happened as mom continued to bring in the reptile to make sure she was doing a good job. "I have to bring Molly in regularly to make sure she is doing okay. If anything happened to her, my son will never forgive me," she said. I told her that she was doing a great job, and it was nice to see that *she* was so concerned for the little lizard.

"I'm not," she insisted.

"Um," I replied. (Of course, she cared about Molly. She kept bringing the lizard to see me when the lizard was perfectly fine.)

"Doctor," she finally confessed. "I love my Molly. Now that my son is gone, Molly is my little girl. I can't believe how attached I've become. Molly is one of my daily joys. She's not only a link between my son and me, she's the reason we talk twice a week. The truth is I truly look forward to seeing Molly, feeding her and I even moved her lizard home into my bedroom."

Clever Molly knew that her family life was changing and decided to finally bond with Mom who had mostly been in the background for most of her lizard life. I wondered what would happen during Christmas and summer vacations, and could have predicted that Mom and son would actually fight now over who would take care of Molly.

I think Mom is winning.

"I call Molly my broach. She sits on my shoulder and we watch TV," Mom confessed, adding, "I sit next to my husband doing this and Molly never moves. But one night, she jumped off my arm and ran to the top of his head. Oh my God, we were laughing so hard! He's also in love with Molly now that our son is gone."

Gotta give it to Molly. She had captured the hearts of the entire family.

Pets do find us in different ways. Some literally wander up to our front door while others are selected at shelters or from those with a new litter of pups needing good homes. If you're going out to select that pet, it is helpful to narrow your search a bit and do some research. Really think about your living situation. For example, I have known some great Pitbulls and I believe they are amazing dogs in general, but they are not my favorite breed because I live in an area with a lot of wildlife. Pits have a heavy prey drive and want to catch things and kill them, which doesn't vibe with my life having a multiple pet household. It's innate in their breed, which means living in a place with so many animals will not be ideal for them or the other creatures who deserve a safe environment.

If I have a client who has a Husky, I'll always discourage them from getting a cat because Northern Breeds (like Huskies and Malamutes) do not mix and it can be deadly to the cat. If you have little children, herding dogs might not be the best pick because they like to bite at your heels, especially if you are running from them. Again, that's who they are – and you need to know your facts so you're not trying to change an animal's innate nature. In a family of two adults, it's no big deal. Kids might be confused by it and say that the dog is biting them, when they're nipping and herding.

You have to accept animals for what they are. If you're precious about your things then a dog that is a major chewer might not be your best idea. German Shepherds are loyal working dogs, but if you don't give them a job then they might drive you insane with barking and nervous energy. The flipside is you don't have to do as much with a Basset Hound who generally prefers to be a couch potato dog. He will just lie around and try to avoid walks. They still need to be walked, but they are very content with just "hanging out." I always feel bad for Pointers who live in apartments because this hunting dog longs to go outside, find birds and point. They're not really bred to be just a pet, but bred to have a job.

The point here is that you need to start your search knowing what pet will work for your unique lifestyle. It has to be more than saying, "It's just such a pretty dog and I felt a good vibe." That's why so many pretty dogs end up at shelters, which is sad and can be avoided if you make sure that the pet in question matches your living situation.

Please do your homework. Use the Internet as a good tool and read stories about people who have that breed of dog or cat. Talk to others who own birds, reptiles and bunnies. Did you know that owning a bird will guarantee you no longer need an alarm clock when the sun comes up? Talk to owners of those kinds of pets when you spot them. Don't get yourself into something you can't finish.

MY VET LIFESTYLE

My days as a vet are crazy and unpredictable, so I like to get up very early to workout and have some peaceful "me time." One brisk, New Hampshire morning, I woke up to find my cats were outside although they're supposed to come in at night. I guess my husband forgot and they spent the evening "camping" and "hunting" in the yard. This wasn't a good thing. Even without my glasses on at the break of dawn, I saw one of the cats had something that resembled a round, furry ball in his mouth – and that "toy" was alive!

It was summer, so there I was in my shorts and tee, running along the wet grass to chase my cat that actually had "found" a baby duck and was holding it within his teeth. A chase ensued and finally, Roo dropped this poor little baby who was stunned and afraid, but thankfully not really hurt. Quickly, I scooped up the duck, did a quick exam right on the middle of my lawn, and then ran it into my house, bolting upstairs.

The duck wasn't stunned anymore and cuddled into my hands.

My husband Andy was actually the stunned one now.

"What is it?" he mumbled in a sleepy voice because for about the ten-zillionth time, I had jolted the poor man out of his sleep with one of my animal rescues.

"What is it? It's a duck," I answered knowing that I didn't have time to tell him the entire story. I was worried that the cat would go and get more little ducks now that I had taken his little play toy away from him.

So, I did what any vet/wife would do under the circumstances. I passed the little bird onto my husband who sat up and said, "Okay, it's 5:30 in the morning and you're giving me a duck?"

"Yes, it will be a great story for our grandchildren," I said. "Take care of him. Her. It. She had a rough night."

Outside again I ran, grabbed my cat and put him in the house. Then I went exploring the yard for a duck's nest. I never did find it, but at least I stopped my cat from hunting at night. As for the little duck, I fixed her up and sent her back on her way although I wasn't sure she wanted to leave. She was already bonding with her new mother….Andy! If we had a pond, I think we would have had a new pet.

To this day, my husband jokes about it, wondering what I will place in his hands next.

Maybe that will be the pet that finds him.

3

Gestalt

I came home after a long day at the clinic with a laundry list of things to do including making dinner and homework. I was at the top of the driveway, only to find that my daughter was outside on her phone. The concept of Mom home was just routine to her although we went through that hurried conversation you have with your kids when they're super busy.

"Hi, Mom."

"Hi, honey."

"How are you?"

"Um."

"What does um mean?"

"Fine."

That is actually a long conversation for a teenager who basically has reached that point in her life where her parents are pretty ignored. (In other words, the way it should be with your kids as they're getting older and finding their own independence).

Same day, Andy opens the front door to our house and my dogs came racing outside, practically trampling me in my process. They couldn't even wait for me to open the car door and practically jumped through the open window into my lap. Once I was on my two feet, they were jumping on me like one of those amazing films where someone is returning home from war. I swear, it wasn't that they hadn't seen me in ten years. They saw me at breakfast that morning. It had been about eight hours in real time that I was gone. Yet, they were deliriously happy to be reunited.

Or as the old song goes: Reunited and it feels so good!

It's a different kind of love with pets that's just completely unconditional and always there. I call it Gestalt, which means an organized whole that is perceived as more than the sum of its parts. Your pets want the whole pack there at all times. When you come home, the pack is more complete and they feel the Gestalt. The whole is whole. It's thrilling that everyone is back at home base. Life is good – and it's time to party by jumping, licking and showing their joy.

Gestalt is a philosophy of the mind where one tries to maintain meaningful perceptions in an apparently chaotic world. The central theory of gestalt psychology is that the mind forms a global whole and that whole has a reality of its own. Gestalt psychologist Kurt Koffka wrote the famous phrase, "The whole is something else than the sum of its parts." Again, it means the whole is greater than the parts. Remember that your pets have this ingrained into their beings. They want the whole.

This theory also applies to healing in animals. Deepak Chopra in his book *Quantum Healing: Exploring the Frontiers of the Mind/Body* also pointed to a study about rabbits with heart disease after (sadly) being fed a high fat diet. The caretaker of one group of specific rabbits who held each one while he fed them had far greater success. His rabbits had a 40 percent reduction in heart disease despite the idea that this caretaker was specifically told NOT to hold the animals. He snuck in that love, showing that healing occurred when the animal felt the wholeness of being part of a loving twosome. They felt the gestalt.

So, what do you do about their joy when the gestalt is realized?

You can easily push them away when they jump on you and knock those grocery bags out of your hands. Yes, it's a bit maddening at times when the cans of corn are rolling down the hallway or when your dog seems so needy that he's practically collapsed at your feet wagging his tail off.

Then again, isn't it great to be part of a "pack" when someone is *that* glad to see you are back on home turf.

Take a moment. Feel the gestalt!

You're lucky if another being rejoices in your presence.

GESTALT IN ACTION

Bosco is a Pitbull, a big and beefy male with a muscular body and a huge heart. He lives with a middle-aged couple, Fran and Jack, whose children are grown and gone. Fran is the first one to admit that she loves Jack, but that Bosco "is the love of my life – just don't tell Jack, although he already knows it's true." Their gestalt just seems stronger as neither feels whole without the other. Her husband can't even get mad because he says the same thing.

"That dog is the love of her life and vice versa," said Jack.

They are a bit confused about how it came to be that their big boy could have so many unique relationships within the same household. For example, Fran can't sit anywhere without having that big white and black head on her lap. Once, she left the bathroom door open a crack and Bosco had his head on the lip of the tub. That wasn't enough for the dog and he even tried to climb *into the tub* with her. Most of the time, Bosco needs to be touching Fran in some way to feel good. Fran doesn't admit it all the time, but she really loves it.

At night, he wraps his feet around hers while he snores at the bottom of their bed. When Fran is out of town, the first thing she notices is that her fur blanket isn't there, and she feels a bit pained, even if she's having a great time on vacation. Back at home base, Bosco sleeps on her pillow to smell her.

Frankly, Jack doesn't get it.

Bosco never does this with him. Ever. Not that Jack would mind, but he has a far different relationship with the dog. Jack is a fix-it type, an active guy who is always tinkering with something around the house. Even when Fran is home, Bosco follows him around, never letting Jack out of his sight. Quite often, he's planting his big furry body just inches away from the action and observing carefully. Jack calls Bosco his "little apprentice" or "fur supervisor."

"I love it because weekends are all about projects for me and Bosco is a guy's dog," Jack insists. "I often feel if he could use a hammer and work next to me that he would do it. But it's none of that cuddly stuff he does with Fran."

Fran thinks he's nuts. "He's just a big baby with everyone," she insists. "Bosco is such a love and just wants pets and affection." Well…that's part of the story. Fran knows, "He mostly wants that affection from me. He's not that into it when Jack pets him for too long. In fact, he will quickly get up and walk away."

"Why does that happen?" she asked me.

So, we explored exactly what was going on with others in the house.

Add one more to the mix. He comes in the form of a spunky and adventurous four-year-old grandson named Manny who comes over three days a week during the summer. It turns out that Manny likes nothing better than peddling his little bike or plastic Batmobile around the back patio. Bosco loves the little boy, licks him, and plays ball with him. But most of the time, he seems to act as his nanny. When the little guy peddles his car, Bosco walks inches behind him. Manny will often get out of the car or off the bike and pretend that he's putting in gas. The dog will either sit at attention or plop down behind the car and just wait.

Clearly, Bosco is making sure that his little charge is A-OK and safe.

This family is typical of many households that have one or several pets combined with more than one person. The truth of the matter is that your pet is doing what he or she is supposed to do in their interaction with humans. The pet is having varied and different relationships with everyone in the household. Just because there is gestalt doesn't mean that once everyone is present and accounted for there can't be different definitions of the relationships within the tribe or pack.

There are intricate relationships between different humans and various animals that prove the sum of any pet experience is so much bigger than the little parts.

HOW YOUR PET INTERACTS IS PERSONAL AND UNIQUE

A family of four finds out that their neighbor's black Lab just had puppies. There's Mom and Dad, plus a girl, 10, and a boy, 12. The family is finally ready to add another being to the mix and adopt a female pup they name Zoe. Mom insists that the kids take over Zoe's care in order to teach them about life and responsibility. It's not long before the boy, 12, has opted out. The girl, 10, is all in. She feeds and walks the dog daily. Their bond is strong and the girl even pours out her daily woes to Zoe.

Three years pass by in a blink.

Zoe and the girl are bonded tightly. They're inseparable and the dog acts as a pillow/therapist/best friend for the girl. The same dog doesn't treat the boy in the same manner. They're buds who play Frisbee and Zoe mostly stays out of his room because he has kicked her out so many times. Mom and Dad love Zoe and she returns the affection, but never follows them around. If they walk in, she's happy to see them, greets them and wags furiously. But then, she just sort of co-exists with them except for when food is involved.

As you can see, Zoe is having four different relationships under one roof. And that's absolutely normal.

In any house with an animal, you won't find two relationships that are exactly the same. You can't even break it down to say that the pup will act one way toward the adults and another way (perhaps more protective) towards the children. Each person and every animal in a household has a unique personality and will interact in a very personal way that will be unique. Your dog won't even have the same interaction with each of your children.

In other words, if you have four kids plus one cat then you have four relationships. Grandma moves in and you add another pet-person relationship, 100 percent different, to the list.

Why does this happen?

I believe that our pets are with us to teach us lessons or fill a need. That's why these unique and different relationships exist. What you need from that one pet might not be what your mate needs. What one child needs is not the same as what the other child wants/needs/will accept. Case in point is a famous actor who adopted three pugs, so his wife wouldn't be alone when he was away on location. The pugs are very affectionate toward him, but seem to have a deeper relationship with the wife including spending far more lap time with her.

"They hardly ever jump in my lap," he gripes.

At night, they never sleep in the curl of his legs, but are virtually attached to her. "Does this mean they don't like him as much?" she asked me, the concern in her voice evident. "I feel bad for my husband because he really loves these dogs, but he seems to get less love from them."

When we looked at the situation, it became clear that her husband really didn't want to spend too much time snuggling with the dogs. He also admitted that he loved the dogs hanging at the bottom of the bed, but didn't get the same comfort his wife did when they curled up with her. At the same time, he was perfectly happy when the pugs did use him as a pillow, which they did when they needed to move positions in bed.

"He's getting what he needs – and you're getting what you need," I said. "It's just different."

The needs of one person or the lessons the person is ready for is taught when the pet knows it is right. The pet connection happening now may be different in the future. A lovely woman brought in Angel, an African Grey parrot who had picked almost all of the feathers on the front of her body to the point that she was essentially naked on her chest. Angel was owned by Francis, an elderly Italian woman in her 90s and her daughter brought Angel in because of the feather loss.

"My mother has owned Angel for 35 years and she has never done this before. She has always been the picture of health. I'm not sure why she would do this now," explained her daughter. After running laboratory tests and determining that Angel was in overall very good health, I started to ask about recent changes in Angel's life that may be causing any stress. Francis's daughter assured me there had been no changes at all. The people in the house were the same as were the food, the cage, and the environment. Nothing had changed. Everything had been the same in her mother's house, just her and the bird for the past ten years since her father died. Even when her father died, the bird was fine.

"Is there anything your mother is stressed about?" I asked.

Francis's daughter sat silent for several minutes, almost not wanting to talk. "My mother's sister died three weeks ago. She would talk to her on the phone every single day, but my mother is very strong. She didn't seem to waver when this happened."

I explained the connections we have with our pets and how sometimes they take on our stress, even when we don't think we are stressed. Francis's daughter sat thoughtfully. She remembered that when her father was alive how he would complain about how her mother always had to talk to her sister each day, no matter what! He joked how she wouldn't know what to do if she couldn't call her sister.

"Do you really think my mother is stressed?" asked her daughter. I told her I thought she should talk to her or maybe call her daily. Several months later, Francis's daughter called me to report that Angel's feathers had grown back in. She thanked me for having her call her mother daily. Sometimes, I feel the gestalt and it is wonderful.

Meanwhile, Vinny, a Great Dane who is 7, lives in a house with three children, a boy, 12, a boy, 8, and a girl, 5. The two younger children are clearly more bonded with the two cats that also dwell there. When the 12-year-old was being bullied at school, Vinny did something I didn't find that curious. Instead of sleeping on his dog bed in the much cooler basement, he began wandering upstairs to sleep at the foot of the bed of the 12-year-old who spent a lot of time in his room crying over his situation. The dog never returned to the basement to sleep.

Not just that one night, but for the next four years.

Different needs require different bonds.

BUT WAIT...I'M THE MOM OF MY FUR KIDS, RIGHT?

Mom. Dad. Brother. Sister. Those are human labels. Our pets aren't walking around with a book to define their relationships in that way. As humans, we want to break these relationships down to the typical household roles.

I'll hear: "I'm the Mom to my kids, so the dogs see me as their fur Mom, right?" Not exactly. Your dogs and cats see you as a loving, nurturing being in their lives who feeds them and dunks them in the tub until they smell like a garden while they might see your husband as the pack leader who keeps danger away. Or maybe you're single and fulfill all the roles for your dog or cat.

Labels need not be included.

For example, I grew up on a farm with a mother and father, but my dogs didn't bond with my mother as their mother figure. In fact, they didn't bond much with her at all because like I told you, she wasn't born a pet person. (The dogs did grow on her, which was amazing to watch). Growing up, the human-canine connection was greatest with me, the child of the house, while the same dogs didn't really connect with my Dad because he was busy around the farm with so many animals. I was their primary caretaker and took on all of the roles including feeding, walking, bathing and loving them. I wasn't their favorite. I was "the main one" in their lives and they were more affectionate with me as a result.

I've had clients come into my vet hospital who have said, "Oh, this is my husband's cat. He's like his Dad and the cat is all about him. He's his leader and I just live there." Or another client will say, "My cat is only about my teenage daughter. I just buy the kibble." In that family, that little brown tabby snuggles with the daughter, but squirms out the mom's hands if she tries to get closer to the cat.

"The cat looks at my daughter as her number one," said my client.

It shouldn't be ranked on a numerical scale either. Mom might not notice, but that same cat greets her and checks on her throughout the day. Occasionally, she does jump up to cuddle, but on her own terms. Looking back, Mom didn't really want a cat, but agreed to it. It seems to me that this cat is giving Mom a full menu of exactly what she needs while she gives more to the daughter who can't go three seconds without the cat in her arms.

Same cat.

Different connection.

It's not right or wrong. It's not good or bad.

Think about the other relationships in your life. Does your brother react to you and your other siblings in the exact same way? Does your Mom treat all of her children with an identical blueprint that feels 100 percent equal?

Instinctually, pets zero in on what we need and give it to us.

Don't ask why your pet acts this way towards you. A far better question is: *What does my pet need and how do I provide it for them? What do I need and how is my pet providing that for me?*

WHY DOES THE DOG LOVE HIM MORE?

Can love be measured? Is one relationship better? You can ask yourself that about both your human and animal links in life.

When it comes to the love factor, I believe that pets give love to all who treat them with love, respect and decency. On the home front, love in a pet is often too narrowly defined by how many doggie licks are given or leaning hugs or cats that jump into laps. There is no need to keep score because that animal is giving you love by just walking next to you or waiting for you endlessly in the window.

Again, ask yourself what you're looking for in a pet. There are some people who love having an animal around the house and are fascinated by taking care of them and observing their behaviors. Others want a more tactile relationship involving snuggling, bonding and that one-on-one we understand each other shorthand.

Does the pet "love" one person more? I wouldn't describe it in those terms. A pet might be connected on a deeper level to one person, but still has a fierce loyalty and love for the rest of the family or pack. Remember that they love "the whole."

WHAT'S IN IT FOR THEM?

There is such a long list of what pets bring to our lives including unconditional love, help with loneliness and depression, and good old-fashioned fun. Petting a dog or cat even lowers your human heart rate and helps you fight high blood pressure.

But what's in it for them? Why do pets choose to live with humans? I believe that animals have a bond with us far deeper than just the fact that we're feeding them and giving them shelter. I believe that they do crave both of those things. Animals look outward and need to satisfy their basic survival needs. Obviously, they need food, water and a place to live. But I believe they also look inward and search for a connection with the humans in their life. That's why they're so intuitive to our needs. They dial into our emotions, try to figure us out and along the way search for opportunities to help and teach us how we should live.

Think of it this way: On many days, you're the grocer, cook and landlord for your pet, but in turn, your animal is your teacher, counselor and little (or big) Yoda spiritual guide.

4

Pets And Affection

I have many hedgehog owners who tell me how affectionate their hedgehogs can be. I often wondered how this could be possible since they were completely covered in spines. Enter a pet named Hazel.

Hazel was a class pet that hid in her hide-away hut most of the day because she was sleeping (they are nocturnal creatures). She had little interaction with the students, so she was not very well socialized. When summer came, my client's daughter, Becca, decided she would take Hazel home to care for her until school resumed. Becca had never owned a pet because her family members were allergic to fur, so she was very excited to have this opportunity to care for her first real animal.

She worked with Hazel every day to get her to not "ball up" when she picked her up. She trained her with treats to come out of her hide-away hut and taught Hazel how to accept scratches under her chin and on her cheeks. Within a few weeks, Hazel began to follow Becca around her house. The hedgehog would sit with her watching TV and would snuggle on her human's chest when she would read before bed. One night Becca had an argument with a friend and she was very upset. She lay on her bed and cried and tears poured from her eyes. Hazel was on Becca's bed "hanging out" and recognized Becca's distress. She licked her tears from Becca's face.

Affection? Love? Connection? All from a hedgehog.

Ever wonder exactly how your pet says "I love you?" Here are some common ways an average pet expresses affection:

CATS

It's all in the tail. When your cat holds her tail high with just a little hook at the end, she is a happy and empowered kitty. There are many felines who will even give a little flick of the end of their tail when they see their beloved humans. But there are several other ways that a cat shows the love including hitting you with his head. That's a way your cat shows friendship to other cats, and quite often that's extended to the important humans in their lives.

Technically, in the cat world, it's a way to transfer their scent located via glands on their heads to others they adore.

Cats also have these scent glands along the sides of their heads and these release pheromones linked to trust, love and familiarity. So, if your cat is rubbing her face against people or certain things, it's a sign that they're in a good mood and feeling the love vibe.

Finally, cats demonstrate fondness with their little mews (a sign that they feel safe) or with half closed eyes and slow blinks (love, love and more love). You can show your cat you feel the same way by slowly blinking back at them. No words needed.

They'll get it.

DOGS

Your dog shows affection in ways that go beyond the standard tail wagging that most of us associate with loving dogs. Yes, that tail wag means things are good, but look at how your dog holds his or her tail at mid-height while wagging like crazy. That means your pooch is truly happy to see you on a heart level.

Other ways your dog shows love is through touch including snuggling and leaning against you, which shows that your dog is happy, relaxed, and trusts you. (This can also mean your dog needs some extra TLC during a storm or fireworks).

Is your dog jumping on your bed at night to sleep with you? It's another sign of love because dogs like to sleep with their beloved pack members including those two-legged ones. Finally, take a look at your dog's face and how he or she looks up at you with an open mouth and those soft eyes. It's another love message as is that leaping up, spaz out greeting you get at the door when you return home …from getting the mail at the end of the driveway!

GUINEA PIGS

Guinea pigs are very affectionate animals that give love when they get love. They will show you affection through nuzzling their head against your hands, or if you hold them close, under your neck. Some will also purr softly if you hold them gently while stroking them. Some will even squeal if they're in a loving and excited mood. They want you to know that they're really happy, so you can share their joy. (This sound can also mean that they need food). Ever see your guinea pig leap up and down in the air? It is called "pop corning" and it means they're especially pleased to see you.

True love is easy to spot with these little animals. There's nothing like a guinea pig licking you as a show of true fondness.

Guinea pigs make up a big sector of my practice. They are extremely affectionate and entertaining little creatures. One such client owns six of these fuzzy beings. She has "floor time" with all of them twice daily. She takes them out of their cages to run around. Most guinea pigs love the freedom to not have an enclosure, but one of her pigs named Mufasa prefers to jump in her lap every single time because he wants head rubs. He even runs to the end of his cage that faces people to get those same head rubs.

LIZARDS, BEARDED DRAGONS AND TURTLES

They're cold blooded, but certainly not cold hearted. Some vets believe love and affection is a controversial emotion in reptiles, but I think that lizards and tortoises do show more emotion to the people they bond with and are quite affectionate with them.

To bring out those feelings, stroke your lizard on the top of his head as this typically makes them happy. Lizards will extend their neck, close their eyes and allow the petting because they enjoy it. Remember that they have a great memory, recognize their owners and really do remember those who show them care and kindness. One note: Bearded dragons love to be held. Put one on your shoulder and they will be very happy. My daughter's bearded dragon hangs out on her shoulder while she does homework. She calls her "my brooch."

Rub your turtles on their shells and they will push into your hand, which shows their joy.

BIRDS

Certain breeds of birds like Cockatoos are very affectionate pets and love to bond and even cuddle with their humans. Other ultra-loving birds include Cockatiels, Conures and Green Wing Macaws. Warning: Cockatoos basically don't stop cuddling as long as you give them affection. Hence the name "Velcro birds" because they like to cling. One does need to be careful with Cockatoos as too much affection will cause long term unwanted medical issues associated with sexual frustration. Be sure to research this before getting a Cockatoo.

Test the waters and see if your bird allows you to pet her on the head. Gently glide your fingers back to front against their feathers. Your bird will let you know if that's okay – or not. Be careful, as bird beaks can pack a punch when they bite.

One of my clients owns Gordon, a green-cheek Conure that travels everywhere with him. He "lives" in the gentlemen's coat pocket, which is convenient for when they travel to the store or to my hospital. When Gordon needs to come out, his dad calls his name and a bird head pops out of his pocket.

RABBITS

Your pet rabbit is a very loving and social animal. He or she is licking your hand for a reason. Rabbits show affection through licking, which is their way of saying that they love you and trust you. Stick your hand into the cage to clean it or give them food and immediately the licking will probably begin. That's a quick, "Love you—and thanks."

This might also happen after you place a hand on your rabbit's head to calm him. They will return the affection with a lick. When out of their cages, your rabbit loves being cuddled and stroked on their head or lightly on their cheeks and will be happy to sit on your lap, which is another sign of attachment.

I never understood how affectionate and loving rabbits could be until I met Sheila. Her "grandmother" brought Sheila to me because her mother could not make the appointment due to her hectic work schedule. Sheila was a jet black, silky, Holland Lop who sat munching her hay in Grandma's lap.

"You must save this rabbit. She cannot die," Grandma said emphatically. "My daughter is so attached to this rabbit. You have no idea."

I didn't know, but I was soon to find out that her mother had escaped an abusive relationship with only her rabbit and no other personal belongings -- just Sheila. That was all …. no clothes, no shoes, no pictures, no phone and absolutely no things. Her beloved pet was truly all she had. Grandma went on to tell me that Sheila's belly was getting bigger and seemed painful.

Sheila had a large mass in her belly that was uterine cancer.

"You cannot let her die," grandma insisted. I was certainly not planning on that, but Sheila had a very aggressive tumor. I was able to successfully remove the mass and Sheila lived for another year.

I was finally able to meet Mom and she told me "You gave me life when you gave her life. She licks my hand every night before bed. I know I am loved. Thank you."

Her heartfelt gratitude for giving her bunny another year to live was so apparent and appreciated.

THE FRIENDLIEST DOG/CAT BREEDS

These lists change all of the time, but if you're looking for dogs and cats that are very affectionate consider these potential new family members:

DOGS
*Labrador Retriever

*Golden Retriever

*Poodle

*Doodles including Labradoodles and Goldendoodles

*Beagle

*Irish Setter

*Boston Terrier

*Boxer

*Corgi

*Cavalier King Charles Spaniel

*Siberian Husky

*Flat-Coated Retriever

*Rat Terrier

*English Foxhound

*American Foxhound

*English Shepherd

*Bulldog

*Basset Hound

*St. Bernard

*Chinook

CATS

*Persian

*Exotic Shorthair

*Abyssinian

*Burmese

*Maine Coon

*Ragdoll

*Sphynx

*Tonkinese

*Birman

*Oriental Shorthair/Siamese

*Egyptian Mau Cat

BONDS OF CARING CAN CHANGE

Can animal-people relationships change? Absolutely. When the Smith family brought home a Golden named Charlie, the relationship between the dog and their young son Ben, 12, was out of a storybook. Charlie and Ben spent all their waking hours together, hanging out in the yard, playing ball and watching TV. Just a few weeks ago, Ben left home to go to college. Yes, Charlie misses him, but the dog still has a lot of love left under that roof.

During all those growing years, Charlie was friendly and loving, but so busy with Ben that he didn't hinge his every doggie happiness on the Dad in the house. "Now that Ben is gone, Charlie won't leave my husband's side," said my client. "My husband is so excited. He always wanted the dog to hang out with him, but figured that Charlie was Ben's dog first. Charlie is now exploring a loving relationship with that pack person who is nearby."

I reminded her that it wasn't a lack of love between Charlie and her husband. It was just a different relationship during the years when it was about a young boy and young pup. But like any union between living creatures, the great news is that it's always evolving. When the son temporarily left home, Charlie created a new bond that has made everyone very happy. He's attentive to the husband, goes on long walks with him, and the two hunker down on the couch for football games on Sunday.

Of course, the minute college freshman Ben walks back into the house, Charlie is slathering him in doggie kisses and they return to their familiar bond based on years of togetherness, but Dad is also in the mix now. Charlie wedges between them for the big game.

Charlie and Dad have also forged their own and very personal new way of interacting with each other and now Charlie has many happy options. I promise you that with one pet there is always enough love to go around. Remember the gestalt!

A BOND WITH AN OUTSIDE PARTY

In a previous chapter, I told you about how animals choose you. They also do this in weird ways including picking you because you're connected to someone else the pet is supposed to interact with in some fashion. You might simply be their avenue to this person, which doesn't mean that there is a lack of love for you or your family. You might just notice that there is an abundance of love for this third party.

Take the case of my cat Roo, a pet I love dearly and one who provides me with all the love back. However, I'd be remiss not to know that Roo has the greatest connection with our nanny. Roo just adores her and the proof is when the nanny walks in the door each morning. Roo can't move his paws quickly enough and runs to her like he's a dog. He even jumps from the floor to her shoulder and perches. The cat won't leave her side and even seems a bit sad when she says goodbye for the night.

"You'll see her again, tomorrow, Roo," I promise and the cat goes on to have a happy night with our family. I just get the feeling that if the nanny forgot her phone and had to run over that the happiest cat in the whole entire world would be Roo.

So why didn't Roo just pick our nanny to be his human? Consider that this wouldn't have been possible. Our nanny's fiancé, a man she has been with for 15 years, is highly allergic to cats. It would have been too complicated (or impossible) for Roo to live with our nanny at her house, so he did the next best thing possible. He chose a way to still be with her during most of the daylight hours. Their meeting was via our family, but Roo immediately recognized this kinship.

It's the same story for a 7-year-old Irish Setter named Max who loves his family (Mom, Dad, 14-year-old daughter), but does warp-speed happy doggie circles each time Uncle Jack comes over to watch football. Uncle Jack travels a lot for work, so he doesn't want a full-time pet. However, Max not only greets him with millions of licks, but does something he won't do with the family. He wedges his body behind Uncle Jack on the couch (not easy since the dog is large) so they are skin-to-skin for the entire game. You can see the euphoria on Max's face. (It's not a surprise that Uncle Jack has a picture of Max on his desk at work!)

When the family went on vacation and Uncle Jack was in charge for a week, Max was delirious with happiness. "Um, no, he's not showing signs of missing you," Jack told the family when they called in to "see how it was going." It was sheer bliss all the way around.

Personally, I think this is a wonderful thing. If someone is bringing great happiness into your pet's life then you should embrace it. It makes their world and yours so much richer.

WHEN ONE PERSON IN YOUR HOUSE IS NOT A "PET" PERSON

It happens. You're the biggest pet person in the world and you fall in love with someone who just isn't "into" animals. Frankly, I do question people who do not love animals, but I don't judge. I'm married to someone who wouldn't have called himself "an animal person" when we first met and we've been coexisting happily with our children and many pets for almost two decades.

If you're the ultimate pet person dating someone who says that they hate dogs/cats/anything furry or scaly then you might ponder if this relationship between the humans can actually work. You'll be living in a house together and you don't want one person to be miserable because a dog is there – or not. I've even heard animal people called selfish for wanting pets, when truly I believe that anyone who loves an animal and takes care of it is selfless.

I digress. There are a lot of people who grew up with parents who weren't pet people. Some of them, like my husband, didn't know what he was missing.

What I actually find quite fascinating is that animals are often intrigued by that one person who really "isn't into them" while the self-described crazy dog lady is the one who gets nipped. Why is this? I believe the animal just doesn't "get it" or can't understand the problem when someone in the house is distant. They feel the disconnect from this person and the animal might be wondering, "Maybe I can persuade this person to like me."

Other animals might perceive this standoffishness as bad energy. Many will look at this person as a "project" and try to win the more distant person over to their side.

I remember my daughter's gymnastics' coach stopping by to drop something off. She was really into my orange cat Crystal, an animal that has a bit of a not-so-pleasant streak. I told the coach that Crystal tends to greet people like a dog would and sometimes even gives someone a little nip. I'm always telling people to be careful and to go slow with her. (We don't want to have one of those "love" bites.) There was that friendly coach, petting Crystal just one too many times, and the cat nailed her! I felt terrible, and luckily the coach was okay with it. In fact, she just laughed it off and said, "I can't understand why any animal wouldn't like me. So many non-animal people I know are courted by their friends' cats and dogs." It wasn't a personal thing. Crystal just had her moods and a very direct way of getting her message across. There are typically no subtleties with animals; we need to accept them at face value.

As for my husband, he is not an animal person. When I met him, maybe that was one of the intriguing things to me. Here was a guy who didn't care for furry things and I was a veterinarian who adored all living things. Like I said, he never had any pets growing up and was quite indifferent to my two dogs when we first met. They were always with me, and he couldn't understand this close relationship.

As our relationship grew so did his with Toby and Cleo (my two Basenjis). He would snuggle with them on his couch and would often take them for walks if I had a very long shift at the hospital. While camping in Vermont, my dogs were being watched by a pet sitter. The gasman came to fill propane tanks and forgot to latch the fence and my two dogs escaped. The pet sitter was able to corral Toby but Cleo was gone. We got the news and our hearts sunk. We immediately packed up our tent and headed back home.

We were both crying during the two-hour drive. By the time we arrived at our house, Cleo had hobbled home with a broken leg. It appeared she was hit by a car. I scooped her up and went directly to my hospital. Luckily, only her femur (the big bone in the top part of her leg) was broken and everything else was stable. It could have been a lot worse.

My husband held Cleo and cried. He was so relieved she was going to be okay after a surgery to repair her leg. I will never forget his words to me: "You promise she will be okay. You promise?"

I knew my dogs had turned a non-animal person into a compassionate pet lover. Before this happened, I was a bit uncertain about having human babies. I always told him, "Until you can prove you can take care of puppies and kitties, we can't have a child."

There were some tough times including when my beloved Toby, at age 20, passed. He had such a special place in my heart even though he was such a naughty little dog!

I wanted to have my very own dog so bad and I researched it thoroughly and decided a Basenji was for me. A breeder was "re-homing" one of his show dogs and gave Toby to me. Little did I know that Toby had bit nine handlers and had a multitude of other quirks. The first week I owned Toby, he chewed up my Coach handbag that I had saved for months to buy! He continued to chew things up during his 20 years including countless shoes, books and paint containers.

One of my favorite destructive tales was when I came home from vet school one afternoon and found feathers billowing down my steps. I quickly ran up to my bedroom and found two Basenji's having the time of their lives shredding my down comforter. My two little black dogs were white because of the large number of feathers they were standing in. In fact, I cleaned feathers for four years!

Toby had a long, beautiful life with my entire family, including my three girls. He adored them because I adored them. When it came time to say goodbye, my husband saw how distraught I was and said, "You love that dog more than you love me."

It was factual in that I had immense love for both of them, and it was factual I did love Toby more, if that is even possible. He had been through college, veterinary school, internships, a wedding, three babies, new jobs and 20 years of my life as my absolute best friend that I confided in over just about everything.

Yes, the love was vast.

Over the years, my husband began to accept and embrace those feelings through so many animals that shared and continue to share our address. There are times he's frustrated and says, "I didn't sign up for this! This is ridiculous. We live in a zoo!"

One of the kids always reminds him, "You knew she was a vet when you met her!"

The other night, I saw my husband carrying around our Chihuahua, Lola. He was talking to her and babying her while she was pressing her small head into his chest.

"Yeah, yeah, yeah," I said, walking past this dynamic duo. "You don't like dogs."

By the way, he's also obsessed with our guinea pig, King Tut, and also talks to him. My husband doesn't clean toilets or do the laundry. Maybe he's wiped down the kitchen table twice in history. But he cleans King Tut's cage twice weekly. Yes, he was really upset when I brought King Tut home after a client brought him in to be euthanized because they could not afford his care. My husband – the one who was not thrilled – still said on that first day with us, "We'll have to get him a much bigger cage. One of those three level ones."

The little pig lives in a pad that's nicer than our house.

My husband would never admit it, but I've turned him. The non-pet person can be found on weekends laying on the couch, watching TV with a dog at his feet and King Tut on his chest.

Not that he's enjoying it – or anything.

My advice with a non-animal person is to figure out their deeper feelings about animals. Make sure it's not allergies that's keeping them from having pets, which is a serious medical concern. If not, test that person with puppies or kittens. All babies are beautiful. How can you not look at a little kitty or puppy and not have an emotional response to it? I think a few non-pet people would be pleasantly surprised if they spent a little time around animals. A day at the local shelter is a good place to start.

Trust Their Instincts

I remember at one point in my life, I was experiencing bad migraine headaches. My dogs wouldn't leave my side. I wasn't surprised that they were so protective and so concerned. Pets have amazing instincts that govern how they operate in the world and interact with other animals and humans.

The easiest way to explain it is your dog, cat or other pet is in tune with nature. While we try to live in the moment, they actually *do*. Their communication isn't based on words that can have several meanings a.k.a. humans trying to talk with each other and add their emotional input, but often talking around the main topic at hand. Animals are pure in that they read energy between beings and then process it through the pack mentality.

In my case with my headache, a member of their pack was sending out the energy that I wasn't feeling well, and the dogs began to hover as protection. Their senses, highly tuned like most animals, immediately kicked in and they came in for what they felt would be the appropriate response to support the ailing pack member.

My headaches passed (thankfully), but this wasn't the end of the interesting ways my own dogs have instinctually communicated with me about something that was wrong.

My dog Toby was quite old when he walked out of an open gate in my back yard at my house. He was pretty senile at age 20. At the same time, I had a small Italian Greyhound, Luigi, who frankly wasn't the smartest dog on the planet. But on the day that Toby – old and pretty unsure of his world – pulled his great escape, the little Greyhound went right into action. He knew the gate was open and raced up to me, barking non-stop, to tell something was seriously wrong. I ran outside with him and we found poor Toby heading towards the road. Thankfully, we saved him – emphasis on "we" – before anything bad could happen.

Animals have a knowing when it comes to something wrong. They're born with instincts, an inherent behavior (just like our intuition), common to all species. Some instinctual behaviors do require some maturation, but evolve as the animal ages. This behavior is often a motivational force in how your animal acts.

Silvan, was a beautiful Siamese cat who lived to 23 years old. His owners have been clients of mine for a very long time. He is an anesthesiologist and she is a nurse. When the cat was a kitten, it would always bother them at night and not let them sleep. The cat would meow loudly and even jump on their heads, thus driving them crazy.

They decided to close their bedroom door and lock the cat out, but that didn't work either. Silvan would just put his paw under the door, grab the underside of the wood and shake it hard. This couple tried and tried to ignore the cat and hoped it wasn't also bothering their young son. Most nights, Silvan was tolerable, but other nights it was incessant meowing.

"What's wrong with our cat?" they said. "We're starting to think that he's psychotic, but just at night. During the day, he doesn't do any of this disruptive behavior."

I knew there was probably a good explanation involving the pet's instinct and the stimulus was only happening at night. Time passed and the couple returned with the rest of the story. One night Silvan was particularly ballistic in bouncing off their bedroom door and meowing a new meow that had not been heard before. They rose from bed to check on the cat, but he was fine. Down the hallway, however, their young son was having a grand mal seizure. All of these "night episodes" with the cat were a loving and wildly concerned animal telling them that their little boy was having small seizures that eventually led up to his bigger one.

The cat was actually the first to know instinctually that something was wrong with the boy. It turns out their son was suffering from epilepsy. On the grand mal seizure night, the cat was so insistent that the couple woke up and checked out the house. They truly believe their son would have died that night without this warning.

By the way, the cat lived until 23 and grew up with the little boy she "saved."

THEY KNOW WHEN SOMETHING IS VERY WRONG

That instinct that something is wrong is deep within your animal. No one really knows how they "know" what they know, or do we? Animals, dogs and cats for sure, can predict seizures in people, can sniff out bombs and fruit at the airport and can "read" the bad guy. How is it done? I believe animal communication works on many levels including pheromones (chemicals of smell and taste), auditory (hearing), visual (sight), tactile (touch) and electric (energy.) As people, we heavily rely on our sight and let our other senses go to waste. For animals, they trust all the cues and process them well when they are needed. This innate ability to process cues, to be aware with lightning fast processing speed, is their instincts at work.

Be sure to listen to that dog whose hair goes up when he sees that person or leads you to a particular area of the house or outdoors. Yes, it's one of those "Lassie" moments, but don't discount it. Your pet might just be saving you from little or big harms just like the lady with the very sweet Boxer who went ballistic one night at the park when this man walked by. The woman even apologized to him for her dog's behavior and the next day read in the newspaper that he attacked a woman a few blocks away the same night. That Boxer knew that there was an energy coming off this man that meant danger.

Research supports the idea that animal senses and instincts are indeed quite fine-tuned. Dogs are being trained now, for instance, to predict diabetic and epileptic seizures. In many cases, they will lay across the laps of their person right before the seizure hits as a warning. They can feel an energy shift is on the horizon. Some believe they can read the "auras" of other living creatures.

What's so interesting is that people who do energy work including Reiki masters believe that animals are like little Reiki specialists. How do they predict? For instance, seizures always have a pre-period where the aura or energy is different. The dogs or cats feel that change, come to sense it and will quite often alert another human being who can help.

As you come to know your pet better try tuning into what they're interested in. It's a good way to read their instincts.

THE GAZE IS CRUCIAL

Perhaps you've noticed that your pet spends a lot of their day just looking at you. Without even knowing it, you spend a big chunk of your time looking at them. This works both ways for a reason according to a team of Japanese researchers who conducted an experiment revolving around the hormone oxytocin, which creates bonding in humans and several other species. Urine samples were taken for dogs and their owners before and after the experimental sessions, which involved the owners petting their dogs, talking to their dogs, but most importantly gazing into their animal's eyes. The findings proved that the oxytocin levels in both the dogs and the humans were higher at the end of the session, but the highest readings were simply from the humans and dogs looking at each other.

It has always been their natural instinct to keep us on lock – and now it's good to know that we're actually de-stressing and upping our own joy levels by simply locking eyes with them.

LISTEN TO THEM

It may help to remember an instinct in your animal is not done by free will or choice. Your cat isn't sitting around thinking, "Yeah, Mom looks a little bummed out today, but I really like this patch of sunshine I found, so forget her. I'm going take a nap." Animals just react to things without even giving it a second thought. It's a reaction to some sort of stimuli that causes them to perform or react in a certain way. Animal instincts are innate, passed from generation to generation, in a pack or breed. They're there for basic survival. Now that you are part of your pet's world, they will also use their instincts for your survival.

Let's say someone comes to the door and your dog is excited. He goes through his routine of barking and running in circles. It doesn't seem to be aggressive, but cautiously excited. That's very typical animal behavior. Then there is the case of the door-to-door salesman that made the hair of a very gentle yellow Lab stand up. I'm talking about all of her back hair standing straight up like someone gave her a punk rock haircut. Consider that the salesman was making the rounds in a suburban neighborhood at 8 p.m., a little too late for this activity. It was fascinating that the Lab's two Doberman friends from across the street were also out walking that night. They spotted the salesman and began to emit low, warning growls. This is an area that gets its fair share of door-to-door, but this one particular man who was out at an odd time had many animals on alert.

What did these dogs know that the people walking them didn't grasp at first? Answer: The guy was bad news. One of the owners asked him why he was bothering people at such a late hour and he had no answers. Another neighbor called 911 and it turned out that the guy was a known burglar who was canvassing the houses for future robberies. In all due respect to the fine men and women in blue who arrested him, I have to point out that the dogs were the first ones who were "onto" this guy. Their warning mechanisms were thrown into overdrive by just sensing him, seeing him and smelling him.

If your dog has that kind of "bad vibe" take it seriously. If they're growling at someone take a step back for safety, but also ask yourself if something could be dangerous to you in this situation. Your pet wants to protect you and is sensing that something is just not right. Choose caution to ensure that both you and your pet don't wander into dangerous situations.

THE JUDGES AND THE JURY

Your pets are natural great judges of character. I have several divorced clients who tell me they should have "listened to their cat or dog" before marrying the person they would eventually divorce. Of course, the flipside of this are the clients who are married and tell me that their dog likes their spouse even better than they like them. Now, that spouse is a keeper!

Your dog or cat bases their decision on feelings that begin with that first impression. There is no waffling. Dogs don't think about it, "Um, maybe I like you. Time will tell, but for now I'm going to go find my squeaky toy." They just know…they're the judge and jury.

Have a party and note what people your dogs or cats gravitate towards and how standoffish they are with others. It's a great way to really re-evaluate your friendship circle!

In fact, I have a rule when I hire people for my veterinary hospitals. If my own dog doesn't like them during the interview, I know that person will never work for me. It says a lot to me when my dog actually loves the person because you truly can't get a better reference from an animal that will quickly size up the situation and give you an instant verdict.

Working dogs are particularly in tune with their instincts, maybe more than some of the fancy designer dogs. Why? They're busy. They have a job. They don't have all day to lounge around and figure it out. They need to make a quick decision and then get back to the task at hand.

I will never discount any animal trying to pass on a message. And I will never get upset with a dog or cat just doing their job and keeping the house safe. It's up to us to listen and check it out. You will never be sorry.

THE CASE OF MY DOG

My Australian Shepherd is a love and prefers kids to adults, but is a friend to all. She is quite sensitive to human emotions and can pinpoint when someone in our family is afraid. I would never expect her to bite anyone or act out aggressively, but you truly don't know how your pet will react when pushed.

One day when I was home with my kids, I had my Aussie next to me outside. She doesn't require a leash and never runs anywhere. Meanwhile, my daughter and I were about to leave in the car with the dog. A serviceman was at our home doing some work and had a big truck parked in our driveway blocking everything. I walked around the truck at the same time another person pulled in. As a joke, he jumped out at us. With the truck there, we couldn't see him and it looked as if someone was jumping out of the bushes to attack us. I screamed and the dog instantly picked up on it and flat out attacked the guy. I couldn't even believe it, but it also wasn't the dog's fault. This person shouldn't have jumped at us. Yes, it was a joke, but I was truly afraid.

This person wasn't harmed, but my dog knew in an instant that I was in the red zone of fear and she just instantly reacted. Luckily, this man apologized profusely and was very understanding (and not harmed too badly). My dog reacted to my reaction in a nanosecond. If I would have not been startled and didn't project great fear, the dog wouldn't have reacted the same way. Let's say I would have realized it was a joke and laughed. My dog would have just wagged away and jumped into our car.

Remember that they're so finely tuned into you that they will act quickly -- especially if you are the one they are strongly connected to and want to protect.

DANGER AND PETS

Out by my pool, we have a free-standing gazebo structure. To stabilize this structure, you are supposed to drill the gazebo into the ground, so high winds won't flip them over. My husband isn't the best at projects, so he skipped that step.

One night, we were sleeping during a really bad spring thunderstorm where the wind actually picked the gazebo up and threw it into our house. We heard a loud bang, but assumed it was in one of the other yards. All of a sudden in the middle of that stormy night, one of our dogs started barking like crazy.

Warning sign number one: This is a dog that never barks.

It was my mini Australian Shepherd Stella who wasn't even emitting a typical sound. Note: I have other dogs that always bark, just for fun, and they were not barking.

My husband and I woke up knowing we had to take this seriously. I was sleepy when I wandered downstairs to find Stella still barking and now growling at what looked like shadows outside.

"What the heck is it, girl?" I asked her. "Is there a huge monster?"

She was warning us that the gazebo crashed into the house and was about to come through one of our windows. Her barking caused us to make sure everyone was out of that room in case the glass shattered. Also of note here is that we have multiple dogs. No one else barked, but they observed pack order, which was that it's the job of only one to provide the highest alert and go find the humans.

These instincts are simply amazing.

When the tsunami hit Thailand in 2004, the animals that lived there just knew. Prior to the actual surge, the birds started to fly away and move to higher ground. Dogs and cats began to flee. Very few animals were lost because they ran for cover. Unlike humans, the animals don't question their instincts. During the recent hurricane in North Carolina, the wild horses that live on the beaches found early places to hide and they all survived. Animals simply think, 'Oh, this doesn't feel good. Run for the hills!"

This proves that animals are actually higher cognitive beings that use their instincts for survival and to make sure that their pack lives on.

YOUR DOG AND THE FIVE SENSES

Let's take a moment to look at how your dog makes use of the five senses:

SIGHT: Dogs do see color, but not complex colors that humans see. Research shows that your dog does see yellow and blue shades, but has trouble with reds and oranges. All in all, your dog has better vision than you do, especially at night when they are especially gifted in picking up movement even with very little lighting.

TOUCH: Puppies enter the world depending on touch and feel from their mothers cleaning them and nuzzling them, the latter of which scientists say is close to a human hug. Your dog's sense of touch is especially sensitive in its paws since they contain nerve endings that even help navigate movement. Your dog's muzzle also has extra nerve endings as does the nose.

SCENT: Your dog has you beat by a longshot when it comes to smelling out a situation. Consider that your pooch's scent area of the brain is 40 times as large as what's happening in the human brain. Dogs are the lucky owners of hundreds of millions of scent-receptors in their noses when humans only have about 400. Your dog spends the entire day smelling like he or she means it, which means with every breath they take.

SOUND: Dogs can hear much better than humans and it informs their natural instincts. In a nutshell, they hear significantly higher frequencies than humans and are also more adept at isolating certain sounds. Even if it's really noisy in your house, the dog will be the one to hear your child fall out of bed because they can separate sounds and zero in on a target of that noise. It helps that their ears are like little mobile satellite dishes, so they can really hear. In fact, scent is your dog's second-best instinct after sound.

TASTE: Humans have dogs beat in this department although your pups will still beg. We have 9,000 taste buds while dogs only have 2,000. That doesn't mean your dog doesn't want to try anything in terms of food. One word of caution: Spicy or rich foods might appeal to them, but their systems can't handle it. Some foods such as chocolate, garlic, onions, coffee, raisins and chewing gum and candies containing xylitol (sugar-free gum and candies) are actually dangerous for dogs, but might taste good to them. Don't give them any of the above.

DOGS AND INTENTION

Dogs sense your intentions. They have an almost psychic ability to sense when something unpleasant is about to take place like you're about to go to the groomer, which isn't always a joyful situation for them. They also seem to know when you're about to engage in mundane daily events such as take a shower (they're running towards the bedroom ahead of you) or give them a bath (the minute you even step outside without the shampoo or a towel, they're running for upstairs). Is your dog reading your mind?

You haven't even looked at the bottle of pills that your vet prescribed. All you've done is stand up and walk toward the kitchen and your favorite feline is running for cover.

Pets navigate the day by reading intentions and closely observing your behavior. A study published in Learning & Behavior found that domestic dogs are as intelligent as a two-year-old human, which is why when you even glance at that pet carrier, your pup is already under the bed. Cats are equally as savvy.

It's the Wayne Gretzky theory in operation. People have studied the hockey legend and one of the things that made him a great player was that he didn't just know where the puck was....*he went to where the puck was going to be.*

He was always one step ahead of everyone else, and it made him a champion. Dogs are the same way, and so are many felines. Your dog is definitely one step ahead of you, watching and listening for the roughly 165 words that they truly do understand. They also can make fast sense of your body language.

Your animals also use eye contact (the gaze) to figure out what people are thinking. They will follow your gaze to determine what's on your mind. Or they just "know" when things happen on a daily basis, which is why they're at the door five minutes before you walk through it. If anyone knows you're late...it's your canine.

Rupert Sheldrake, English author and biologist, is currently studying dog's telepathic powers in predicting when owners arrive home from work. His work shows that dogs can anticipate their owner's arrival despite not having cues and owners arriving at different times everyday. His work is quite controversial, but I believe it to be cutting edge and very poignant. He believes dog's anticipation is dependent on telepathic influence from their owners.

I have always believed, prior to Sheldrake's work, that your pet knows when you are about to walk into the house because your dog is using his sixth sense or intuition. Pay attention to it. If there is something we could learn from our pets, it's to become more aware and follow our instincts and perhaps communicate with them through telepathy.

TRUST YOUR INSTINCTS ABOUT YOUR PET

It's up to you as the human to provide your vet with the most complete and up-to-date medical information about your animals. There are times when you must tell your veterinarian when your instincts conflict with the diagnosis.

Very early in my career, I was working in an animal emergency hospital, which was very busy that night. A young man with a baseball hat came in with his Akita who was quite well-behaved and calmly sat next to him. It was the man who was quite distraught while the dog looked perfectly healthy.

"Something is really, really wrong with my dog," the young man insisted.

The technician showed him into a room right away and I examined a dog that looked normal upon our initial physical.

"I'm not finding anything on my examination," I told the man who shook his head.

"Listen, there is something really, really wrong with my dog," he said.

"Okay, I believe you" I said. "We'll do blood work, x-rays and urinalysis."

"You need to do it right now," he said.

I completed the tests and found through the X-rays that the dog's intestines were filled with significant gas, as was his entire abdomen. When the bowels fill up with gas it presses on the largest blood vessel in the dog's body and shuts off blood supply quickly. This condition (intestinal torsion) is sadly marked by the death of a dog. We usually discover it after the fact and during an autopsy. It's almost never diagnosed on a living dog because they die from it that quickly.

This young man was right. His dog was seriously ill and we rushed his Akita into emergency surgery. After untwisting his intestines, removing his spleen and removing a tennis ball from his stomach, the Akita made an uneventful recovery. This dog survived and was perfectly fine a few days later, but it would have been a far different story if this man wouldn't have insisted that we take the extra steps.

No one knows your animal like you do.

I always listen to owners. It's a case of Mom and Dad do know best.

This Akita taught me early on that human companions need to go with their guts. If you think something is truly wrong with your pet then you're probably right. I wasn't as experienced in those days and could have missed this fatal condition. Again, if we had not acted immediately, the dog would have not survived. Later, I talked to the young man while his dog was sleeping peacefully in recovery and said, "How did you know?"

"I could just tell that he wasn't himself," he said. "He wasn't acting normal. I knew something was really wrong."

A STORY THAT STILL MAKES ME SMILE

One of my favorite stories about dogs and instincts began with a client of mine who had a chocolate lab mix named Nick who had heart murmur. The owner was an engineer who worked tons of hours, so I would make house calls to check up on Nick. Nick was feeling healthy and he seemed stable, but we had to be sure. I recommended a cardiac ultrasound to determine what kind of heart disease Nick had. There was just one little problem.

"Doctor, could I even ask you to pick up Nick and take him to the ultrasound," my client asked.

"Of course," I said.

I wasn't really sure of the route between Nick's house and the animal hospital where the ultrasound was taking place. I didn't know the speed limit in the area either. All of a sudden, I was doing 55, about 20 over the speed limit. There were flashing lights behind us, which Nick found really stressful. He was always the nervous type, and now he was panting like crazy.

I wasn't that happy either because I knew I would be getting a speeding ticket, not to mention, be late for the ultrasound appointment.

The officer tapped on the window and I rolled it down.

"License and registration," he said.

"Listen," I said. "I'm a veterinarian and I have a really sick dog in the back."

By now, a pretty healthy Nick was standing on the backseat vibrating, shaking and panting with nerves from those spinning lights. "I'm on the way to the animal hospital because I think this dog is going into heart failure and he needs an emergency procedure."

The poor police officer looked at me and Nick who sensed this was a time to play it for all that it was worth. He fell off the back seat like he was collapsing or fainting. The concerned officer said the magic words, "I understand. I'll run back to the car and give you a police escort there."

When the officer walked away, I shut the window and Nick popped up on the backseat wagging.

"Nice job, Nick" I said.

We made it to the animal hospital in record time and the officer even offered to help me carry Nick out of the car. I took one look at the backseat where a perfectly fine dog was again shaking because the policeman rattled him. I was the one who picked up Nick and ignored his loving kisses as I carried him into the hospital. After thanking the officer, he left and I let Nick stand. He happily ran around with the staff before his test.

Nick, whose heart was so big that it literally touched his chest walls at one point (when it should have been the size of a softball) went on to have his ultrasound and lived to be 18 years old. His owner was so good about making sure he was at every appointment and gave him his medicine on time.

About one year prior to Nick's passing, a board-certified cardiologist asked me if Nick's X-ray was that of a dead dog because his heart filled his entire chest. She did not think it was possible for Nick to be living. I assured her he was and doing well. Nick's heart was big in so many ways.

By the way, I never did get that speeding ticket!

Later that day, I told his happy owner, "Nick did well today and I have a story for you."

Animal Communication

As humans, we use words to make our needs known. Animals make use of other means to get their points across to humans and other animals while listening to the verbal commands that we make a part of their daily existence.

As a cat owner, you know for sure that your feline understands when you say, "Don't jump on the counters." Your dog also knows precisely what you mean when you tell them to stop begging at the table *right now*. There aren't many pets who don't understand when you say the word "treat" and come running. Most also understand the word "no" even if they choose to ignore you after you say it.

Animal/human communication is a two-way street. Quite often your pet can express in a few bits of body language exactly what they want and need from you. A scratch at the door means, "I have to go potty -- pronto." Standing over the water bowl while looking at you intently is a good indication that it's empty and they want that drink. A bunch of licks on the face means, "I'm so happy that you're here."

Researchers are quick to point out that animals are gifted with various special ways that signal their wants and needs, plus feelings.

Human language and communication is considered exceptional and complex but I believe we can learn a wealth of knowledge from our animal counterparts.

Be on the lookout for these signs:

Auditory Communication: Your dog lets out a bark to go outside. Your cat stands there meowing when she's hungry. It's the same way that birds chirp and wild coyotes howl to signal their needs. Verbal or auditory cues are a way for your pet to get his or her point across in their own verbal way. Animals use a lot of different sounds to communicate from your dog's low growl that a stranger is approaching to your guinea pig's little yips when the food bowl is being filled. It's usually pretty easy to figure it out although with certain animals, it's sometimes necessary to rely on your veterinarian to determine if that's a cry of pain or perhaps separation anxiety about you leaving the house. It's worth a quick check to make sure everything is good.

Tactile Communication: Your dog leans into you for a "hug" or your cat rubs up against your leg and starts to purr. Your dog sits at attention and then throws you an obedient paw. Those are all ways your pet is using their tactile skills or the power of touch to tell you what's going on with them in the moment. Consider that in nature mother tigers lick and nuzzle their young while chimps groom each other. In domesticated animals, touch might be used for comfort, to establish dominance and even establish bonds of trust and caring. Dogs will put their paws over your hand or some will jump up on the couch and insist one body part on them touches your leg or arm. That's your animal checking in and finding their safe spot.

Visual Communication: Animals are quite visual and use how things look to express their needs, wants, and feelings. Basically, your animal is looking for visual signals as active creatures that are navigating their day.

Perhaps a visual to them is you jumping into bed at night. That's a visual signal that the day is over and they're going to sleep. Another visual might be that moment each morning when you reach for your car keys. That signifies to them that you're about to leave for work and they begin to get restless and then bark.

Visual signals are key when you're walking your dog as they can sense and then pinpoint danger up ahead. Pay attention to what your animal has in their scope and use that information to inform you about the world at large. Visual signals also tell your pet when your car pulls into the driveway or when your son returns home from college and your dogs and cats become very excited.

Our pets often use a combination of auditory, tactile, visual and instinctual cues to communicate the world around them.

HOW TO TALK CANINE

You might not want to admit it, but most of us frequently talk to our animal companions. I'm no different because I greet them, tell them a bit about the day and even say goodbye or goodnight to them. You may think it's a one-sided conversation, but it's amazing that certain pets (perhaps all) seem to know exactly what you're saying to them.

In my hospitals, I insist that my technical staff talk to the pets before we do procedures on them. For example, if we are drawing blood on Fifi the dog, the conversation goes like this: "Fifi, I am going to draw blood on you today. I am going to use the vein in your back leg and my friend is going to hold you and give you love." As crazy as this may sound, we have little objections from our pets.

The truth is they do understand when we verbally communicate with them. They even understand when we do not verbally communicate with them. Perhaps they don't know every single word, but they grasp our meaning and emotions. If you're riled up and talking about how that contractor is running late, your pet knows your frustration. The flipside is when you're vacuuming singing along to ABBA, they know it's a really happy household and a pretty good beat! Perhaps they start to run around like crazy and celebrate your joy.

Scientists estimate that smarter breeds of dogs and cats can learn about 160 words. That's not nearly enough, so you can make use of other ways to make your pet know exactly what you want in the moment.

Visualization is a technique that truly does work because animals are visual creatures. They create images in their minds based on what you're saying at the time.

Try this quick exercise: When you speak about a certain topic, visualize it through pictures in your mind. Think about it for a few minutes. Your animal will pick up on the image while listening to your words. In fact, you don't even need to say the words. Think of yourself as a projector sending your image to their minds. If you're really clear about your image then the animal will understand better. Be precise.

For example: I need to find my purse, but don't know where I last left it. Visualize the purse as you talk about it. You will say: "Where is my purse" while still thinking about it. Your dog might be the one who actually finds it.

This works in other ways. Let's say there is a sock on the floor. You don't want your little puppy to grab it and maybe try to eat it. Your mind is visualizing that sock while you try to outrun the dog and grab it. In a crowded kitchen that dog zeroes right in on the sock and grabs it. Why the sock and not something else in that kitchen? You've visualized it so much that you've sent the message out. Now, it's a big game of chasing the dog to get that sock. In other words, your dog just had a really fun time….and you two have certainly communicated!

You can try visualization during playtime. Go outside and say, "Get me your red ball." Maybe there are six different balls on the lawn, but you clearly ask for the red one while thinking about just that red ball. You've asked your dog to fetch and they're clear about this desired action. I'm guessing that the dog will race out there and grab that red ball.

THE CONVERSATION BEGINS WITH YOUR EMOTIONS

I can't really think of a dog person who has to tell their canine, "I'm really scared." Let's say you're walking at night and there's someone who looks like trouble just ahead of you. It's not necessary to put your dog on high alert because he or she knows in the way you're suddenly gripping the leash harder, breathing a little faster or sending little stress signals out. Your dog knows that you're afraid. You don't need to put it into words, which is the magical thing of having an animal in your life.

It's not that they're reading your mind…or are they? They're reading your signals: gripping the leash, breathing and walking faster, and maybe even making a call in a nervous voice. This is communication. . .They may also be reading your mind. According to Sheldrake's survey of pet owners in England, 46 percent believe in their pet's psychic abilities.

Just be careful what signal you put out to your animal. One of my clients told me that it was hard to walk her Lab because she barked at all other dogs, but never humans. Each night, they would go out and it would be a barking festival with her apologizing to all the other people walking their dogs. When she married, her husband took over the nightly walk and …guess what? The barking stopped. Same dog. Different reaction.

The truth was the woman always gripped the leash tight and went into DEFCON Five mode each time a new dog walked by. The husband talked gently to the dog and gave the command "focus" each time a different dog was in their path. It got to the point where the Lab was out there smelling other dogs and making friends for the first time in her life.

If you give dogs the reason to tense up and react, your dog will take you up on the offer. Same thing applies to the doorbell ringing. Does your dog race to the door barking like crazy or calmly walk to the door with you? You might act tense anticipating their barking, which in turn feeds them and creates the frenzy in the first place.

The truth is most of us (thankfully) are never put into a true life or death situation. If you're creating tension remember that your pets will be able to pick up the subtle scent of your adrenalin. They will quickly learn to associate it with fear and danger – and act accordingly.

One afternoon, my nanny was watching my three girls at my house. It was on the day the local high school does this prank that the seniors call Suicide. They try to capture someone by stalking other seniors. It's all in good fun, and thankfully my kids were much too young to participate.

That afternoon, the seniors mixed up our house with another. Two older boys burst into our backyard (instead of our neighbor's yard). My nanny and the girls heard the commotion and were really frightened. Meanwhile, my dogs were inside, but when these two big guys pressed their faces to the back door, it not only scared my children and my nanny, but also the dogs went into action.

My 20-pound Aussie was attacking the slider door and aggressively barking, feeding off the communication of fear from my terrified children.

I was actually happy that the lines of communication were so open. First, two big guys shouldn't be in my backyard ever, unless invited. My dogs did exactly what they should do after picking up on those non-verbal cues.

Dogs will spring into action and race in for the rescue with the small canines following the lead of the dominant one. The signs are there that your dog is about to flip that switch: Back hairs stand up, pupils dilate, lips curl and they have a change in stance. This is what I call fear posturing.

They know you're afraid…you don't have to say a word.

REMEMBER THEY COMMUNICATE ACCORDING TO THE PACK:

It's a good time to remind you that dogs communicate according to the pecking order. Dogs rely heavily on social hierarchies to determine what they are and are not allowed to do (or say) in a setting. Dogs live in the military-like system, everybody in the unit reports to the alpha (or commander). Canines do what the alpha dog would do or want them to do. Alphas go through the door first, eat first and lead the way. Many dogs will let the alpha communicate more with the humans. It makes sense. The alpha is their leader, so it's up to him or her to bark out the orders – pun intended.

COMMUNICATING WITH CATS

Cats have very finely tuned senses, and communication with them is pretty simple, sometimes. The first thing you should notice is your cat communicating with the swish of her tail. If her tail is straight up and curled at the end then she is happy. If she is twitching her tail a lot your cat is excited or anxious. If her tail is almost vibrating then your cat is really thrilled to see you. Watch out if the tail fur on your cat is sticking up straight up or they curve that tail into the letter N. This is an extremely angry cat that can become aggressive. A fight might be on the immediate horizon between two cats. But, if your cat's tail fur is sticking up, but they're holding that tail low, it means that your cat is scared.

Another way to communicate with your cat is to look directly into her eyes, which is not only a bonding experience, but a way to "speak" cat. One warning: You must blink or the cat will think you're doing this as a sign of anger or aggression. A cat whose pupils are dilated shows they're in a playful mood. The cat staring back into your eyes means trust. A cat that slowly blinks is communicating love.

Let's say you tell your cat to stop climbing on top of a cabinet. Your cat is staring at you, but now tilts his or her head. This is your cat saying "I get it" or "I acknowledge you." Cats will often wait for you with that stance, which says I am waiting to see if you will follow through. Same cat that slicks his or her ears back either feels anxiety or is ready to play.

Other cat communications:

*Rubbing against you means that you belong to the cat.

*A wet nose kiss means the cat enjoys you.

*Hitting you with the cat's head means the cat is being playful and affectionate.

*Rubbing his or her head against you means affection.

*Small licks are a sign of major trust.

*A cat bite means another one is coming. Back off.

You can communicate love back to your cat by giving your cat little eye blinks. It says "I love you." Hold your cat in your arms while you do this and you will find that your cat will become calm and relaxed.

Also speak to your cat with a low voice as their hearing is quite sensitive. Yelling loudly doesn't really work because cats hate shrieking voices and loud noises.

A FEW COMMON CAT SOUNDS DECODED

What is your cat telling you?

*Meow. They need attention.

*Purr. They are content.

*Between a Meow and Purr. A happy greeting.

*Growling. Leave me alone or this will escalate.

*Hissing. I'm angry or scared.

*Yowling. A fight is brewing.

YOUR CAT KNOWS GOOD CHARACTER

This is a story of a little tabby that didn't like her owner's boyfriend. When he came over, the cat would attack the boyfriend's shoes and hiss at him. "Is my cat telling me who to date?" my client asked me. My response: "Your cat is telling you something. She's communicating and I would listen to your cat because they're much better judges of that deeper inner self, which sometimes we don't easily, clearly or want to see."

We see something else. Cats pay attention to the real core.

A year later when she came back in for vaccines and a check-up, my client told me that she broke up with her boyfriend…and not because of the cat. "He was a bad guy," she said. (The cat called it!)

MAKE SURE IT'S NOT MIRRORING

Sally comes home and she sees pee on the floor. She stands over the pee and says in an angry vocal tone, "This is horrible, you cannot pee in the house!" The dog lowers his head like he's really feeling bad. "He feels horrible about it, but still does it," Sally told me.

"Did you stand over the pee and talk in a low voice? Did you sound very serious?" I asked her and she nodded.

If you did, the dog is just mirroring your emotions. They're not communicating in your terms, they are empathizing or matching you. You're upset, so they will be upset.

Another example of this is when I meet clients with rescue dogs. One had a dog that was beaten by a previous owner. "He is soooo nervous," my client said.

The reality was the dog has moved passed this horrific situation and, more times than not, it's the new owner who has such remorse mixed with anxiety over it. The dog seems anxious because the new owner is anxious. It's not that he is having flashbacks of his prior life. Remember that dogs (all animals) live in the moment. They are not humans that carry baggage around with them. They move past terrible trauma. Dogs can have "trained responses," but they are not wallowing in their abusive past. Some of you may disagree and say "I know my dog remembers!" Remembers what? They can certainly remember because that is how training and cues work.

Let's say your dog is in your bedroom. An earthquake rattles the city and the floor vibrates. Your dog becomes very scared and he may not want to set foot back into the bedroom again because of the conditioned response. Does that mean your dog will NEVER go in your bedroom again because he sits all day long worrying that the floor will quake again? No, your dog doesn't want to go in your bedroom if you are trying to make him because that is where the floor quaked. However, you can re-condition him to go into the bedroom with training and positive reinforcement. Dogs and cats don't think and worry about the past. They only have conditioned responses based on the world's cues and current situations.

Rule: Your pet doesn't dwell mentally in the past. Your pet wants to be in the moment, and your pet wants you to be in the moment as well.

YOUR VET COMMUNICATING WITH YOUR ANIMAL

As a veterinarian, I can be an internal medicine doctor, a radiologist, a surgeon, an ophthalmologist, a psychologist and a dentist, but I cannot be a mind reader or look into a crystal ball. No one can look into that swirling ball (except perhaps a psychic) although there is a spot in veterinary medicine for animal communication.

Danielle MacKinnon is a gifted animal communicator who has written two books and appeared on TV and various radio shows. She taught me that in veterinary medicine, we are limited because the animal communicates with us and sometimes we miss what they're trying to tell us. In fact, animal communication bridges the gap between what the animal is trying to tell us and how we interpret or misinterpret the data.

For example, a client tells me that her dog is constantly eating rubber toys.

After a scary blockage, we tried to examine why the dog does this all the time? Is it out of frustration? Do the toys taste good? Or is it because the dog isn't getting enough attention? You have to look for the clues and try to communicate with your animal through body language. Yes, we found out that this hopeful looking dog, after racing for her leash two or three times, and the owner not going on that walk would then go over to his toy pile and eat something out of frustration. Or so it appears.

That is the label we give it: Dog wants to go out for a walk, the owner resists, thus the dog is "mad" and eats a toy. Or is it something different? The dog wants to go for the walk, doesn't get the walk, so now he decides the next best thing is to play with his toys and destroy it because the dog enjoys it.

Which scenario is it?

Increasing the daily walks from one to two actually changed the behavior, but we still don't have the answer to the question. Yet, the animal was clearly communicating through actions and a chain of events. We still don't have the clear answer as to why.

This is where an animal communicator can really help us. When I have a situation that I can't fix, I look to experts in the field or alternative fields to find answers—even if it seems a little "out there." Animal communication is a very useful tool when I have exhausted all of my medical knowledge and the pet still does not have a diagnosis.

Penelope is a Lutino Pearl Cockatiel who once had beautiful feathers. Her owner came to me for "feather picking," which is an extremely frustrating condition for owners because their beautiful birds pull out many or all of their feathers and it's hard to figure out the cause. Penelope had pulled out all of her feathers on her chest, back, legs and neck. She still had feathers on her wings and head, but was now essentially a naked bird.

The first step was a medical workup to rule out underlying medical causes. After all of the diagnostic tests were found to be normal, I diagnosed Penelope with behavioral feather picking, meaning I had no idea what was causing her to pull out her feathers. We tried Penelope on medicine to relax her, but the problem persisted and actually became a little worse. The owner and I talked at length about the living conditions. What changes had she made? Were there any new pets, people or changes in the household? We tried to figure out what may have set Penelope off, but everything had stayed the same. I then recommended she seek out a reputable animal communicator.

She did.

The animal communicator told the owner that Penelope was feeling wind under her cage and it bothered her feathers. The owner went to investigate and noticed that there was an air vent below Penelope's cage that had always been closed, but for some reason was now open. My owner closed the vent and covered it with a thick towel to make sure no "wind" bothered Penelope.

Within six weeks, her feathers grew back. I'm thankful that Penelope is fixed and fully feathered and that the animal communicator solved the feather picking.

AN ANIMAL COMMUNICATOR TO THE RESCUE

I have seen animal communicators help with medical problems, but I was also privileged to be a part of finding a missing dog with some very special help. A client that bred dogs named Julie was placing one of her agility dogs, Harley, in a home in Connecticut. The dog was high energy, a great runner and had quite a bit of zest in him. He loved to bark and run the agility course. An active woman in the agility circuit named Angela was very excited to have this two-year old dog become part of her family pack.

Angela picked up Harley from my client in New Hampshire and drove to Connecticut. The next morning upon entering my hospital, I had a message to call Julie ASAP because there was an emergency. She was hysterical because when Angela arrived at her house in Connecticut, she opened the hatch of her SUV, unlocked the kennel and tried to place the leash on the dog's collar. Something startled Harley and he bolted off into the woods. Angela searched all evening for him, but could not find him. She called Julie who jumped in the car hoping that if she called for him then he would come. Julie was on her way to Angela's house when I called.

"I don't know what to do," Julie cried. "How am I *ever* going to find him? Angela lives next to *hundreds* of acres of conservation land. And you know how Harley can run!"

This was all very true. Harley was an extremely agile dog with great speed. I knew he could really be anywhere in those hundreds of acres or even could be trying to run all the way to Julie's home.

"I know this may sound crazy, Julie," I told her. "But another client I know is an animal communicator. I can ask her if she will do an emergency session with you to help you find Harley."

It was really the only thing I could think of in the moment. Julie was desperate and readily agreed.

I called the animal communicator and had her contact Julie. It wasn't long before she had some interesting information as to what Harley was communicating directly to her. The message: He was deep in the woods and couldn't move. He was looking at a big clearing of trees with a grassy knoll where there was a white house. It was very foggy.

Julie had no idea what all of this meant because she was driving, but when she arrived at Angela's house she asked about a grassy knoll with a clearing of trees and a white house. Angela responded that it was on the other side of the conservation land, but it would be very foggy over there in the morning. Julie was so excited when Angela told her it was foggy—just maybe she was onto something.

Angela drove Julie to the white house and they walked and walked over the grassy knoll in all directions. The forest was very thick, but Julie made her way through it while calling for Harley again and again. Finally, they heard whining and rustling in the woods, Julie quickly walked toward the whining. She could barely make out Harley who was stuck in the nettles, but when she made eye contact with him, the dog barked like crazy!

Once Julie and Angela were able to cut him out of the nettles, they turned around to walk back to the car. Julie immediately remembered what the animal communicator had told her—*he was looking at the clearing of trees with the grassy knoll and the white house.* Well, this was exactly what she saw when she turned around. She simply could not believe it. Julie called me on her way home to share the "great rescue story."

It remains one of my favorites.

DO ANIMALS REMEMBER?

One fascinating aspect of animal communication is wondering if they remember the past. As humans, we hold on to the past and have deep emotions that stay connected to what happened yesterday and all the days before. I believe that animals move beyond it and want to live in the moment.

It is truly beautiful that they can live this way.

Have you ever wondered why your dog greets you with great enthusiasm every single day when you get home? Answer: He is in the moment-enjoying the reunion. If your dog doesn't greet you, and he typically does, be concerned. Your pet might be ill.

By looking at animal communication, we gain many lessons as humans including: Let go of the past; live in the moment; embrace your power; trust that you are being taken care of in each moment; and finally, our beloved pets are here to teach us-we must be open to receiving.

Your Pet Is Your Mirror

I'm a firm believer that our pets choose us for a reason. They're here to teach us a lesson or show us ways we can improve our own lives. We help them; they help us. It goes both ways. In fact, it goes a little deeper for most pet-human relationships. That's why I say that your pet is your mirror. Much like we look into a mirror to check how we look, our pets are looking into our hearts and souls to show us what's going on inside of us on a deeper emotional and physical level.

Take the case of an owner I'll call Nancy who is a very anxious woman. She came in to see me about her very anxious dog named Winnie. "This dog is crazy. She can't sit still. She's just running around the house all day and never stops. It drives me nuts," Nancy said. Meanwhile, I'm looking at her (the woman) and thinking, "Wow, you're pacing around our exam room and playing with your fingers, ripping at your cuticles, talking to me *and* checking your phone. Now, who is it that can't sit still? Who is the anxious one here?"

It's easy for me to pinpoint exactly what was happening here. Winnie was simply mirroring the human's behavior. When the woman calmed down for a few minutes, the dog took that as a cue, curled up in the corner of the exam room, took one of those big, fill-your-tummy-with-air sighs and took a little nap.

It's hard to say what came first? The chicken or the egg? Was the dog nervous first or the human? My vote is the owner who is a nervous woman by nature. Winnie has learned how to mirror her behavior. Of course, perhaps the dog was a little anxious to start by nature, but just revved that up to 10 after living with a very emotional owner. Chicken or the egg? That's a question you can never answer.

Or can you?

One of my clients, Sara, lost her beloved pet and swore she would NEVER have another dog the same as her Shelby. Shelby was a Golden Retriever that stayed by her side while finishing college, getting her first job and having her first baby. Several years later, Sara was ready for a new dog and was very interested in a mini-Aussie.

At the same time, another one of my clients bred mini-Aussies and had one she was trying to place in the most loving home, her four-year-old retired breeding dog. Sasha was a relaxed, quiet and loving dog who was a great listener and loved to snuggle. Sara met Sasha and it was love at first sight. Several months later Sasha had become very anxious. She was barking at "everything" and Sara was worried she would bite someone.

We met to discuss Sasha's behavior, as she was a different dog from her early days. Now, she was very "on guard" and "unsettled." After multiple diagnostic tests, I determined that Sasha was medically sound, but behaviorally changed. Further discussion with Sara yielded insight into her life. Sara had been a stay-at-home mom, but since her son had moved on to high school, she decided to start working outside the home again. This was very stressful for Sara because she felt she could not balance being a mom for her son and being a dedicated employee for her new boss. Sara was very frazzled, constantly on edge, and in Sara's words, "I am not who I want to be."

The dog was mirroring Sara's behaviors. Sasha had been a very quiet, relaxed pet in her previous home, but now that her owner's life and home environment was hectic and stressful, Sasha was becoming a mess.

It took some conscious "calming down" to return Sasha to her former state. Even Sara realized that if this stressful environment had continued then Sasha would have probably been better at another home. Sara didn't want to lose the dog and made adjustments.

One thing is certain: Your pet is telling you what YOU look like in the world.

Another patient told me about her mixed breed shelter dog who hated when the doorbell would ring. The dog would take a sprint for the bedroom and hide under the bed. Funny thing was the woman was sick and tired of these "aggressive door-to-door predators," as she called them, pounding on her door and would run upstairs in order to make them think nobody was home. Maybe the dog ran faster for shelter, but it was basically the same behavior. Doorbell equals go upstairs and hide! One fit under the bed while the other slipped into the bathroom.

The flipside of this is the sports loving guy who has a bulldog named Norman. "Norman is about the laziest dog in the entire world, Dr. M," he told me. "All he wants to ever do is sleep on the couch, get up, eat, drink and then go back to the couch."

The ironic part of this is that the owner during football, basketball, baseball and every other season of sports lived the same way when he wasn't at work. He would stay on the couch in front of the TV, eat, drink and nap.

The dog was simply his mirror.

Same thing for the woman who lived on the beach and never wanted to come inside. Her little dog bounced out of bed (like the owner) each morning for their big walk and spent the rest of the day on the terrace upstairs soaking in the sun and sea air. Both were extremely athletic, sleek, lean and ready for the next adventures.

Two mirrors and a beach house!

HOW DO YOU HELP YOUR DOG?

Perhaps you're happy with what your dog or cat is mirroring. But if you're not satisfied with the behavior, the first step is to do a check up on yourself. If you have one of those nervous dogs, it helps to look inward and ask, "Am I an anxious person in life?" If the answer is "yes," you might follow up with vowing, "Maybe I need to look into some stress relieving techniques." That nightly walk that you extend to 45 minutes might be good for both of you.

If you're gaining weight and the dog is chunking up, it's time to look into how you lay around, which also makes your pet into an inactive creature that will pack on the pounds.

So many times, I'll actually say to an overweight pet owner with that overweight pet, "Do you walk your dog?"

"Do I look like I walk my dog?" I've heard. "I just open the back door and say, 'Go in the yard.' The dog runs out and is back inside in three minutes."

"Do you eat pizza?" I'll ask.

"Yes."

"Does the dog eat pizza?"

"Yes."

Once again, your pet is your mirror. You're living a sedentary lifestyle with high carb snacks and both of you are gaining the weight.

It's helpful to look at what's really going on with your pet by asking, "What's going on with me?" Then you might have to admit, "Some of these issues are truly my issues." It's not uncommon for the mom who barks orders at her kids from downstairs to have a dog who just likes to bark at everyone. Again, it's a case of the dog mirroring the human behavior.

It's true. They're taking on your issues as you transpose them onto the pet. That's why so many times, I'll say, "The problem with the pet is the problem with the person."

Ashley has a Rottweiler. She's a friendly type who stops and talks to everyone while the dog meets the neighborhood dogs. It's not a mystery why Annie the Rottie is beloved by everyone from the mailman to little kids. Another family on the block has a Rottie named Henry. His owner is always yelling, "Don't go near my dog. He doesn't like people." The owner growls at all that approach and so does the dog who feels his master's tension and reacts in the same exact way, but without the words. The intentions are the same as are the end results.

RX FOR YOU AND YOUR PET

The mirroring is not only on an emotional level but also on a physical level with medical problems.

Remember Zoobiquity and how animals and humans intersect? We share the same diseases, and sometimes our pets mirror our disease. This is perhaps the level of connectedness I see that amazes me the most. This is where our pets teach us to better care for ourselves.

Princess was a nine-year-old cat that was not feeling well. Mom had just moved up from Texas and had not been able to find a veterinarian because she had been dealing with her own medical issues. Princess came to see me on an emergency visit and after running blood tests, I had very bad news for the owner. I explained to Mom "Princess has an extremely high white blood cell count and this is very concerning."

Mom stopped mid-sentence and asked me, "How high is the white blood cell count?"

This was odd because most owners do not care "how high" a white blood cell count is.

"Are you in the medical field?" I asked.

"No, I am not, but I have a high white blood cell count," she said. "It's 80,000, and I know what that means."

I paused in shock and continued, "Princess's white blood cell count is 79,000."

Mom burst into tears. This high of a white blood cell count in cats (and humans) can be indicative of cancer throughout the body. Mom knew this because she was experiencing the same thing. In the end, Mom and Princess faced their battles together.

The mirroring of medical conditions is a very common occurrence that I see. I sometimes feel like I can fill in the client's sentence. I will deliver a diagnosis and the client will immediately say, "I have the same thing."

It happens all the time.

I have a client named Ed who is a professional athlete nursing back a debilitating muscle injury in his leg. It wasn't long before he brought in his Labrador Jake who was also limping.

Several months later, Jake needed a tooth removed because it was abscessed. So, did Ed! Finally, Ed was having terrible stomach problems. You guessed it. So, was Jake. All were malady mirrors that were resolved when Ed paid attention to his issues and Jake's issues.

I can't tell you how many times I see animals manifest the same physical issues as their beloved humans. The dog ruptured his cruciate ligament in his knee. The owner said to me, "It's so weird. I just blew out my knee."

Another client didn't look well (the human) and I asked her what was wrong. "I have these chronic bladder infections," she said. The odd thing was her cat was also having lower stomach issues that I diagnosed as a bladder issue. I told the owner this and she couldn't believe it. Or I'll diagnose the pet first and the owner will tell me that they're having the exact same human medical issue. I'll hear, "I totally get it. I have that, too."

What is the explanation? Do our pets manifest our disease? Do we do the exact same things as our pets to produce disease such as eat poorly, not exercise, and perhaps expose ourselves to toxins?

What is the answer?

I believe that pets manifest our conditions as a way of telling the humans to take better care of ourselves.

Many diseases begin with stresses on the body including chronic inflammation. It's easy to see how an owner and a very observant pet can experience the same stresses – maybe not for the same reason – but the pet picks up on the owner's stress and internalizes it. Many pets eat what we eat, which isn't always a good thing, but creates the same medical conditions, especially in the stomach region.

Did the pet have it first and then the owner gets it? Or did the owner get it and the pet manifested it? I believe that these issues usually begin with the owner, and the pet is the mirror to show you what is happening and then acts as an understanding companion by your side *living it with you as both of you get through it.*

THE MYSTERIES OF THE MIRROR

Occasionally, I'm stumped on how a human and pet can mirror each other when it comes to physical illness.

Mark, a construction worker, brought in his indoor cat Shelley who was pretty sick. "She has had diarrhea for two weeks," he told me. "She's never outside. We live in an apartment. She's my only cat, and I already changed the food." Shelley didn't seem to be getting any better. I ran a fecal test and found that Shelley had giardia, a parasite from an outside water source.

"It's a little strange for the cat to have giardia when it usually only comes from outside sources and not the tap," I told the owner. Luckily, it was treatable with medicine, but Shelley kept getting it again and again. She could not clear the infection.

I started doing some research and found that some indoor cats get giardia from their owners. I called Mark back and said "I don't want to be too personal, but do you have constant diarrhea?"

"I didn't want to mention it doc, but I do," he said. "I've had it for about two months, but I hate going to the doctor."

I insisted that he go and get his poop tested to see if he had giardia.

He tested positive. "Does your cat drink out of the toilet?" I asked.

Bingo! It turns out that Mark had been drinking bad water from his construction site and Shelley kept drinking out of the toilet and became sick herself. Had Shelley not become ill, Mark told me it would have been very unlikely that he would have ever gone to the doctor.

I'm happy to report that both are fine these days. Mark brings bottled water to work and Shelley doesn't go into the bathroom!

The point of the story is that pets and their people are so closely linked that they mirror both the physical and emotional traumas of everyday life. When you live with an animal, you're adopting a very similar mindset. It's like a famous line from the show "Outlander" when Jamie says to Claire, "Don't worry, there's two of us now." Your pet is thinking that 24-7. There are two of you now: Mirrors of each other!

WE ARE PET DETECTIVES

Yes, you have to go a bit Nancy Drew when you're a veterinarian.

This is why owner input and honesty is so important. I find that with my owners that sometimes "over-share," I collect the most important and pertinent information.

It was closing time at the hospital and a frantic owner called because her chameleon's body was convulsing. Our receptionist had her head right down. When she arrived, her chameleon was in a covered shoebox and mom was very upset because she had never seen her chameleon exhibit such odd behavior.

My technician went right in to assess the situation. She opened the shoebox cover and saw the chameleon in a hunched position contracting her body and actively laying an egg. She immediately closed the shoebox cover and instructed the owner not to open the shoebox and that I would be right in.

Chameleons are reptiles that are difficult to breed in captivity. It is not common for chameleons to lay eggs, especially those that are not housed with male chameleons. Reptiles lay eggs, just like birds, and if the male reptile does not fertilize the eggs, they do not hatch and they are not viable. There are many reptiles that will lay eggs in captivity without the presence of a male reptile. Female iguanas and bearded dragons will do so often and sometimes even become egg-bound because the right conditions to lay the eggs are not available. The right conditions include the female reptile having optimal nutrition, the right substrate (like sand) to dig and bury the eggs and optimal humidity and temperature. This chameleon in the shoebox did not have optimal conditions to lay the eggs, but she was doing it anyways.

I went in to talk to the owner and explained to her that her chameleon was actively laying eggs and that we shouldn't disturb her and allow nature to take its course. In addition, I explained, "I believe she will be fine once all the eggs in her belly are laid."

"How can my chameleon be laying eggs? There is no male chameleon!" she asked. I went on to explain how reptiles can lay eggs even without the presence of a male reptile but the eggs would not be viable. She then asked me "Is this like pseudo-pregnancy?" I paused, because this is not a typical question from an owner. Most owners have never heard of a pseudo-pregnancy. Pseudo-pregnancies are most common in dogs and cats. They will exhibit all the signs of pregnancy including weight gain, belly swelling and lactation, but they are not pregnant. Some will even have labor signs.

"Yes, this is essentially a pseudo-pregnancy in a chameleon but true pseudo-pregnancies are seen in dogs and cats," I said.

The owner quickly added "and in people."

"Yes, pseudo-pregnancies are also seen in people," I agreed. My owner went on, "I have a pseudo-pregnancy. Is it related to my chameleon?"

Now, as a veterinary professional, I try to maintain a straight face all the time ......but this time, my owner noticed how I was staring back at her.

"You look surprised," she said, adding, "I'm scared. Can I catch this from my chameleon?"

"No, no you cannot catch this from your chameleon but your chameleon may be mirroring your symptoms," I said. "It is possible."

Never had I had a more dramatic display of a pet mirroring their owner. The owner and I talked some more and she explained what it was like to believe she was pregnant, feel like she was pregnant and not be pregnant. It was devastating to her because she wanted a baby so badly and she had to live with the symptoms, but not with the true process of a real life growing inside of her. I knew this could last for nine months and not result in a baby. In humans, a pseudo-pregnancy is considered a psychological and hormonal disorder that requires psychotherapy and counseling.

In our pets, we have never thought it to be a psychological issue, but a hormonal issue exclusively. This made me think that we may actually have it all wrong—a true pseudo-pregnancy in our animals may be similar to that of humans. In humans, doctors are really unsure of what "sets off" a pseudo-pregnancy, but they do believe it is an intense desire to have a baby. Do our pets have the same affinity to reproduce? Do they want an offspring to love and care for? I had never thought about it until this owner walked through my door and told me of her devastating news. Just like her pet, she even looked pregnant, felt like she was carrying a child, but didn't have a fertilized egg growing into a fetus.

Once again, our deep connections with our pets teach us about ourselves and that same connection can tell us about our pet.

It's a mirror, a reflection of ourselves, and a type of self-awareness that gives us pause. We experience, they experience, they learn, we learn. It is a conscious or very mindful relationship for your pet; we need to pay attention to them.

Don't Stress Them Out

This is a tale of two dogs. One is a Doberman who races up to the front door and growls when someone dares to ring the doorbell. It's not exactly a coincidence that this protective boy named Henry lives with a bachelor who hates to be bothered. "I worked all day. My home is my sanctuary," said my client Todd who adopted Henry from a breeder. "I live in a neighborhood where there's always someone coming to your door trying to sell you something. The minute I hear the bell ring, I get angry and sometimes even let out a choice word."

It's not surprising that when Henry was a puppy, he made the connection: Doorbell rings – ding-a-ling- and my human gets MAD! This human I love walks harder and faster to the door and sometimes he's yelling. As Henry grew into an adult dog, his working breed instinct kicked in and told him, "I'm here to defend the roost from this intruder. When Todd goes into defense mode, I'll be right by his side running and barking. Team Todd!"

It turns out that Todd's stress over this issue has rubbed off on his four-legged friend's life.

Megan is 30, lives alone, and always feels vaguely uncomfortable when workmen have to enter the house to fix something. She has a tiny Maltese named Dixie who doesn't like workers either. Megan was worried because Dixie would always run into the corner or under the bed and shake when these people were in the house. "She doesn't do that any other time," she told me. Yes, it was a different response from big, tough Henry, but it was the same cause because our animals pick up on our emotions.

Your stress is their stress.

Without knowing it, Megan was putting off a vibe to Dixie that shouted, "Danger! Intruder! We have to get out of here!"

I asked Megan if her own behavior was a bit different when workers were around and she searched her mind. "I know it's not the politest thing, but I have this habit of pacing around in another room until they leave," she said. Little Dixie began to put the triggers together: Worker plus pacing equals a little doggie panic attack.

It's fascinating how the animals mirror exactly what the owner is feeling in the moment. Emotionally speaking, it doesn't matter if you're a being with skin or fur, two legs or four legs. When you're giving the stress signals then your pet is thinking, "Problem! There's a problem!"

So many times, I see wonderful pets that have a series of behavioral issues because of owner-induced stress. It can come in the form of shaking, hiding, barking or even a persistent licking of the fur that causes sores. It can even manifest physically into a sick stomach. My first move is to wonder, "What's going on with this owner?" because this dog or cat is so distraught over what's happening in their world, which centers on the human.

Quite often, I've been asked if our fears rub off on our animal companions. Think about it for a minute. If you tremble during a thunderstorm, it's no wonder that your 150-pound Great Dane is hunkered down hiding in a dark closet. You might only have a slight reaction of fear, but your pet is going for survival.

Science has shown that dogs can see, hear and smell the signs of human emotions, says Biagio D'Aniello of the University of Naples, Italy. D'Aniello and his colleagues tested human sweat when they were shown fearful, happy and neutral videos. The fear sweat was exposed to dogs and they showed more stress when smelling fear sweat then neutral or happy sweat. The study showed that dogs smell your emotional state and adopt your emotions as their own.

I grew up petrified of the dark. I could never sleep in the pitch black and I needed a nightlight for many years. Even now if the house where my family sleeps is really dark, I'm a little nervous and I'm the grown up. If I'm in the dark and one of my dogs gives a little bark, my startle reflex will kick into gear or I might mouth, "What is it?"

I've noticed that one of my smaller dogs gives out that little fearful woof signaling she's afraid, too, but only after my reaction. Dogs, especially, have that pack mentality that dictates, "Let's all be freaked out together."

So, what comes first? A nervous owner or a scared pet? I often think that the people do come first and pass on their anxieties and emotional stress to their pets. Most pets operate from a general rule that high levels of anxiety are not part of their world.

"Am I making my pet crazy?" my client asked.

It wasn't the first time I fielded that question. I wouldn't go that far, but it is good to keep an eye out for your triggers and try not to involve your pet in them. A client of mine was going through a nasty divorce which meant several heated phone calls. She noted that her dog would cower when she raised her voice. Instead of continuing this, she decided to step aside and take a walk while talking to her lawyer. A walk without the dog. It fixed the problem.

It's funny that pets actually train us on how to exist together.

Let's go back to that dog that barks incessantly when the doorbell rings. The owner doesn't open it, but over the barks screams out, "I'm not interested! Go away! I don't accept solicitations!'"

All the dog is thinking is: "Mom is stressed, so I'm stressed. I'll be barking at the stranger while my human is yelling, which is like barking. Yay! We're doing our job of protecting the house together! This is so fun!" If you don't want the dog to bark, you might need to change your own behavior instead of reinforcing bad habits.

I know many owners who give treats to their dog after barking when the UPS guy arrives. The dog gets extremely agitated the minute he hears the zoom of the truck coming down the street. Clearly, they are reinforcing this behavior by giving the dog a treat every time it happens. Any behavior that is reinforced will be repeated. If you do not want the barking when the UPS man shows up, be sure not to reinforce it by treating it.

Let's say you're at an event with your five-year-old child. You want your little boy to be quiet, so you bribe him with candy. In fact, you keep giving your son candy to make sure he stays quiet the entire time. You're basically saying to this little boy, "If you even attempt to be loud, you'll get a candy to shut up again." It's the same with pets. Reinforce a bad behavior and it will continue.

Any behavior that is reinforced will be repeated.

OUR MODERN TIMES AND PETS

In today's day, everyone is so busy on the phone. We spend a lot of time pacing around the house, doing 15 things at once. Your pet is observing you all the time – and all that pacing and body language when you're figuring out the cable bill is taking a toll on your animal. He reads that as you're mega stressed. Your voice is different. Bolder. Higher. You're not walking lightly, but hard and on your heels. The dog might start running around or bark when you're raising your tone.

"Why does my dog bark when I'm on the phone?" I'm asked.

Why not? You're upset; they're joining the stress party!

If you sat down on the couch or in a chair then your pet will sit with you and maybe even take a nap. If you're up looking like there's trouble then their stress meters go off and they're up and going into action. Think about it: Your pet is stressing out just like Mom or Dad.

Another area of stress for our pets is the pet obesity issue. Over 50 percent of our pets are overweight (for dogs and cats) and we are to blame. Most of our pets cannot reach their food, so they rely on us to feed them. Many of us are overfeeding pets or giving them food instead of the attention and care they really want. For dogs and cats, most think every meal is their last meal. They have not learned (although some have) to be selective with eating. Many clients will say, "Look at his sad eyes…he wants a treat." For me that often translates to this: "My dog looks sad. Let me give him a treat so *I* feel better." The act of treating a dog is to reinforce a behavior we want to see again and not because it will make us feel better. Instead of feeding your pet more and more food for you to feel better, try giving them love, affection, attention and see how both of you feel!

Pet obesity, human obesity, and eating disorders are what I see as psychological disorders of the mind that manifest into physical ailments. Learning to control your pet's diet and to feed your pet for the sake of "keeping them alive and healthy" is very different than feeding them because it's fun to do. Food is a fuel. It is meant to provide sustenance and nutrition. As people, we confuse it with fun, enjoyment and often a replacement to make us feel better. By feeding our pets properly, we can learn to eat with control and remember the true purpose of food.

This is an area that has really impaired our pets, especially our cats and dogs. By overfeeding and feeding the wrong foods, we make them sick. We do the same exact thing to ourselves. The power of the mind is truly incredible—it can talk us into and out of things in a split second. It doesn't always make the correct choices. Try to make the correct choices for your pet and then try to apply those better choices to your own life.

SEPARATION ANXIETY

Many dogs stress out because they have what we call separation anxiety. It's a very real condition because these dogs and even cats don't want to be alone.... ever. In one case, a dog had such a severe case that he would monitor his owner in the morning. The minute the man reached for his car keys, the dog began to bark because he associated keys with leaving. The man had to go to work and just put up with his dog barking upon his exit from the home.

These types of dogs need conditioning work to desensitize them from the idea of being alone. You have to reinforce with them that although you do go to work, you always come home.

Take the case above. The man should reach for his car keys and then go out to get the mail and immediately come back. Or reach for his keys and then go in the backyard and come back. If he does it repeatedly over a period of time, it will reinforce in the animal that reaching for car keys and leaving doesn't always mean such a big chunk of time gone.

Separation anxiety is a very difficult behavior to understand and treat. I highly recommend working with an animal behaviorist or a veterinary behaviorist to help understand the problem as well as treat it.

Look for the cues in dogs with this type of anxiety. Many breeds are very smart and log your routine into their minds. Reaching for the vitamins might signal leaving. Or maybe it's when you open the newspaper. Your dog is one step ahead of you here, so it's helpful to shake up your routine, so they don't have cues certain.

Figure out what the cue is and switch it up. Birds are also very good at picking up on these cues and can be easily trained or ill-trained – take your pick.

Before I became a veterinarian, I worked as a veterinary technician in an animal hospital. Every Saturday and Sunday morning I would go in early to let out the boarding dogs and clean cages for all the pets that were boarding at the hospital. One dog that boarded every weekend was named Max. I felt bad for Max because he was at the kennel every single weekend. I would let him out first and let him run around the hospital a little bit extra because I didn't want him kenneled so long. Just before the hospital would open I would call, "Max! C'mon Max! Come here Max!" Max would kennel up.

Boarding every weekend along with this pup was an Amazon parrot named Zeus who was in the same area where Max would run around. Zeus and Max would interact through the cage bars and almost seemed to become friends. Zeus's vocabulary was very good. He would tell me, "Hello. Watcha doin'? Go to bed. Take a nap. Love ya. Zeus. Bye, Bye." These were just a few of his words.

After months of boarding, Zeus's owner chatted with me while dropping off Zeus for his weekend stay. "Do you know who Max is?" the owner asked.

"Max who? Does he work here?" I wondered.

"All week long, Zeus says to me, 'C'mon Max! Come here Max!' He won't stop."

I paused and started laughing; I had trained Zeus to call Max (the dog) when Max wasn't even there. I asked the owner "When does he do this?" The owner replied "Oh, it's only when I start putting things away in the morning and just before I leave for work."

So, here is a bird that was trained by my cue when I was calling Max back to his kennel. While Max ran around, I'd put things away. Zeus linked that to mean: In the morning when you pick things up, you call for Max!

Our pets learn from our cues, even when they pick up things we don't intend them to internalize. But they do.

STORMS

Many of my clients ask me how to deal with their dogs during thunderstorms.

I even have clients whose Poodles won't put a paw pad outside if it's even lightly raining. I have a fenced in backyard and I direct my animals right out that door, rain or shine. They've learned that if it's raining, you go out, you pee fast, and then you run inside. I only wish I could teach them to wipe their feet!

My Italian Greyhound is the one who really freaks out at rain while the rest are fine with it. Luigi can't get his feet wet. He would rather recline on the couch all day, holding it until the end of time, if it's raining. He did this all day once and then seemed to pee for two minutes straight at night when the storm passed.

Thunderstorms are a different thing because of their electrical pull. Animals feel that electricity in the air and it can really upset them. If you have an anxious dog, he will even become your weatherperson because he will sense that storm coming and stress in advance. You're not imagining it. The dog does feel the atmospheric change.

The best thing to do is to put that kind of pet in a safe room in the house either down in the basement or even in a bathroom with a lot of copper piping because then they won't feel the pull of electricity as strongly.

Many pet stores sell what's called "thunder shirts" for pets to wear. They look like little straight-jackets and fit snug to the pet. I think they do work for some animals. There's also Rescue Remedy, made of several flower essences including Rock Rose (to alleviate terror and panic), Impatiens (to mollify irritation and impatience), Clematisto (to fix inattentiveness), Star of Bethlehem (to ease shock) and so on. It's sold in pet stores. A few drops in a pet's water or under their tongue also help certain dogs. I believe it works in mild cases.

You want to make sure in severely stressed dogs that they don't jump through a window during a storm. Some will do that in order to find a safe spot if they can't locate one in the home.

Your job is to make that safe spot. I know a large Bernese Mountain Dog who climbed in her mom's closet during storms and hunkered down over her shoes. He liked the smell for some reason and felt calm in there. Make sure it's safe for the pet and allow them to remain in that spot until they're ready to come out.

In these cases, there is not much else you can do, but wait until the storm passes.

A note about cats during storms: Most don't show their anxiety because cats have better Chi. They're cooler about the whole thing. The cat is thinking, "Yeah, I know there is a storm. But are you serious? Is the dog really hiding in the pantry?"

STRESS RELATED MEDICAL ISSUES

I have noticed a trend in cats that have stomach upset. First, I would like to clear up a misconception that it is normal for cats to vomit all the time, IT IS NOT. Cats should not vomit unless they need to get something out of their stomach, like a hairball or something that did not agree with them. If your cat is vomiting daily or even 2-3 times a week, please see your vet. The trend I have noticed is that cats that eat more processed, dyed foods with grains in them vomit more and have more skin problems.

Preservatives, dyes and grains cause inflammation. Cats are carnivores and are meant to eat meat (they are actually meant to eat the whole mouse but most owners would object to feeding this) and our processed cat foods don't help with digestion. In fact, they often cause chronic inflammation, which leads to chronic vomiting. The grains (including wheat, corn, rice), the synthetic preservatives and the colored dyes cause stress on the cat's stomach and intestines.

Many cats that are on these diets loaded with grains, preservatives and dyes will develop inflammatory bowel disease—much like humans. This inflammation in the stomach and the intestines will lead to inflammation in the pancreas and then cause pancreatitis in our feline friends. To fix it, we must eliminate the stressors that are causing the inflammation, which will make the cat feel better. This means feeding a minimally processed grain-free food with no dyes and no preservatives or natural preservatives.

Cats are not the only pets that suffer from inflammation caused by stressors. Lick sores on dogs are a good indicator for any vet that your dog is stressed or maybe bored. Certain breeds will just lick and lick until they create nasty deep wounds that need to be treated before they are chronically infected. As I deal with the medical part of the wound, I always ask the owners, "What kind of stressors are there in the home?"

Most people look at me like I'm crazy and just want me to bandage their dog's leg and give them medicine to fix it.

"That licking is a way for your dog to comfort itself. It's like a pacifier," I'll tell them. "It's actually an OCD-like behavior."

Dogs make these lick sores because there is a problem at the site where they are licking. Maybe their leg hurts or maybe its itchy. It's difficult in many cases to know the inciting cause, but oftentimes once they start on that site, they cannot stop.

Sometimes, it's easy to figure out the trigger for the animal. Your bird is picking at himself when you leave the house for long periods of time. Or your dog is feeling ignored because there's a lot going on in the house.

I had a case of an Amazon bird named Tuna. I had vetted Tuna for what seemed like forever. He had no feathers on his entire body -- just feathers on his head and wings. I did a series of blood tests and various other laboratory tests only to find that on the inside, he was perfectly normal.

I believed Tuna's issues were behavioral or emotional, but I could not pinpoint what was the trigger. The client did not return for a while, but the next year, she brought in Tuna for his annual checkup. Wait! Tuna didn't look anything like that featherless bird.

"Oh, you have a new bird," I said, looking at my new "patient" who was covered in gorgeous feathers.

"No," said my client, laughing. "I got a divorce, moved into a new apartment with no yelling to live in peace and my wonderful bird grew all his feathers back. We've never been happier."

Again, what was stressing the owner was causing her bird to pluck out his feathers.

Cats are also quite emotional to stress in the home and can even lose their fur and develop psychological alopecia. They will clean themselves repeatedly in an OCD way and lick off all their fur if they're in a stressful environment. Or perhaps you've seen a cat with all the fur licked off one leg or his or her belly.

I had a cat owner whose feline friend only did this in the hot summer months. I performed a big medical work-up including multiple blood tests, X-rays, urine and fecal tests. I noted that each September, all of the cat's hair grew back.

It happened several summers in a row. Finally, my client told me that every weekend, but only in the summer, she would leave and go up to her lake house. The cat saw her owner leave every Friday, while the cat stayed home alone with enough food and water for the two days, and a neighbor peeking in twice a day.

You didn't have to be a detective to figure out that the cat was sad or stressed when the owner left and chewed off his fur.

Remember that veterinarians are a bit like detectives. You have to give us the most accurate information and all the details because our patients can't talk. When I say to "tell me everything," don't hold back.

You also have to remember to seek medical answers that go beyond stress, remembering that stress and pain go hand in hand for animals.

A woman who owns three Boston Terriers came to see me because the oldest dog, 12, had chronic skin issues. We had always been able to control it with medication, but it was getting worse. When she brought the dog to me, it was really bad. All the hair was missing on her ears and her feet were chewed raw. The owner felt absolutely terrible.

I did a skin scrape and fungal tests and found out the dog had ringworm. Ringworm, isn't really a worm, but a fungal infection that is not that common in dogs, especially older dogs who rarely go outside. Upon examining her other two dogs, they were also affected.

"Do you have a cat?" I asked.

She didn't have any cats, which was key because dogs rarely get ringworm, but cats do. Then the woman said that she had been feeding a feral cat on her back step. The dogs frequent that step daily although never when the cat was around. In the end, the dogs all had ringworm from the feral cat hanging around the yard.

It's important to rule out medical issues like this one before just blaming the entire licking on a stressed pet.

WHAT SHOULD YOU DO TO DE-STRESS YOUR ANIMAL?

Stop. Look at your own behavior.

You might say, "But doc, I'm just walking my dog and she's going crazy each time we pass another dog." Are you really just casually walking or are you on danger patrol. Maybe it's you who sees that dog half a block down and begins to tense up on the leash. That's like a one-way ticket for your furry friend to notice that mom is stressing. Red alert! You're giving the "Danger, Will Robinson" signal by doing something that might feel like just a move to bring your pet in closer and protect them. They freak out more because it's a big world and they don't just have to defend themselves, but they have to save you, too.

The opposite of a pet defending you is exhibiting bad behavior in the house due to stress. You might have a cat that will pee in inappropriate places and not in the litter box. Perhaps this happens at certain times, but not at other times. The cat will hear mom and dad fighting and act out by peeing, but when all is quiet he goes in the litter box. It is called inappropriate urination in cats and often is stress related and can be any stressor from emotional to medical. Figure out the cause and the cure can be found.

My own dog, Cleo, taught me to look at my own behavior. Cleo was a sweet female Basenji that seemed to have some quirky personality traits. One of her aggravating behaviors, at least for me, was that she would dig non-stop at the corner of my couch every evening around five p.m. It was like clockwork. Sometimes, she would have a toy bone to bury. Other times, she would have nothing. This persistent digging would happen when I returned home from work and tried to get dinner started. Meanwhile, there was much chaos in the house upon my return with my three toddlers.

Back to Cleo who would incessantly dig and dig and dig at the corners of my couch. I would yell, "Cleo, STOP!" and she would pause for a brief second and then go back to digging. I would physically go over, pick her up, take her off the couch, tell her to stop, and she would immediately jump back up and start digging. Out of frustration, I placed my toddlers in the corner of the couch, so Cleo would stop digging. Cleo would dig over the girls, while the girls giggled, but Cleo would not stop.

Finally, I sat down in the corner of the couch and Cleo settled and laid down. This was my only solution. As long as I sat and did nothing, Cleo was calm.

It would be several years later when I understood what was going on with Cleo. For my birthday, a friend gave me a gift, a session with an animal communicator. I had never even heard of an animal communicator and wasn't sure what they actually did. I learned that animal communication was a way some people are able to know and understand animals.

My first animal communication session was with Danielle MacKinnon, a gifted animal communicator. The session was on the phone. Danielle introduced herself and asked me if I had ever had a session like this one and I told her, "No." She instructed me to not tell her anything about my pets except their names. At the time, I had two dogs, Toby and Cleo, my Basenjis. She also instructed me to only tell her yes or no if the information she was giving me was meaningful. She didn't want me to offer anything else but that yes or no.

She paused quietly for several minutes and started my session.

"Toby is a big dog in a little body," she said. "He is very proud of himself and has no confidence issues. He likes to come to work with you because he is much better behaved than all the other dogs. He also likes your three girls and likes that they dress him up."

"Yes," I said.

"Cleo is much more nervous and a bit standoffish. She doesn't like how fast the children move, but she really likes it when you sit down on the couch," she said. "She wants you to sit on the couch because all of the commotion makes her nervous."

This was all shocking to me. She had nailed Toby's personality. She knew I had three girls and she knew they dressed him up! She also was spot-on with Cleo and her personality. She did genuinely enjoy when I sat on the couch.

I had never met Danielle, my friend had never met Danielle and no one, except my family could know this information. During a 50-minute session, I was stunned by the information she gave me. There was no other possible way she would have this information unless my dogs were truly communicating with her. But how?

I don't want you to say: "Okay, Dr. Magnuson, now you are talking crazy... you really think she was talking to your dogs?"

Yes, I really do believe she was communicating with my dogs. Please read on.

Albert Einstein was a great physicist of recent times. He is known for his theory of relativity and he shifted the beliefs of science when it came to understanding what occupies space. His work with others like Newton and Bohr added to the study of quantum mechanics. This is the study of teeny tiny particles of energy we cannot see. It is how X-rays were discovered and developed. Now there are oodles and oodles of equations, documentation and belief that radiation (X-rays) exist. I use them every single day in my practice. I send a beam of radiation through a patient and somehow, miraculously it shows up on my computer screen. It happens in a matter of seconds. I rarely think about it, but I accept it as true and factual because it is repeatable.

Particles of energy are everywhere. We cannot see them, just like we cannot see the radiation when an X-ray is produced. We don't think about these particles but somewhere, somehow, someday, someone (who understands quantum particles more than I do) will explain these different energy worlds of love, intuition, telepathy and psychic ability.

Have you ever been thinking about someone that you haven't spoken to for a long time, talk about them to a friend, then surprise—they call you the very next day? It is not a coincidence; its energy. We don't have to understand it to enjoy the rewards of it.

This is how my relationship with Danielle MacKinnon started. I wanted to know and understand how she did what she did, so I took her classes, attended her workshops, and learned animal communication from her.

This is how I learned that in order for Cleo to get the chaos to stop at 5 p.m. in my house, she would dig in the couch. It would always get my attention and get me to sit down and be present with my family. This is a behavior I should have adopted when I got home from work, but wasn't doing. She taught me how to do this—and how important it is to be present with your family when you have been gone for eight hours!

Thank you, Cleo.

Here's a scenario I see all of the time. You have a dog that is shaking, essentially vibrating in the vet's office, whimpering and crying. The owner has brought with him a little Ziploc bag full of treats. The nurse brings both into a room and I'll walk in, pet the shaking dog and the owner will slip the animal a few treats "to make him feel better."

This is exactly what you *don't* want to do. What the owner is doing is reinforcing the animal's anxious feelings. It's like you're saying, "Sam, here are some treats. I applaud you for your little nervous breakdown each time you see the vet. It's fine. Anxious is good. You get treats for stressing yourself into a quaking mess."

"This began in the car," the owner says. "We only go in the car on the way to the vet."

Why not make going in the car a fun thing? Sometimes you go to the pet store, sometimes you go to the park and sometimes you go to the vet? Mom or Dad is pretty much the same no matter where we go. In the vet's office, the humans sit on the bench and they're pretty chill. The dog will think, "I'll be pretty chill, too."

It's just another stop.

DEALING WITH SADNESS

I thought I might mention how pets cope with human sadness. Just like stress, dogs know when you're sad. They pick right up on it and adjust their own behavior accordingly. Perhaps they might act more subdued or gently rest their head on your lap. They will even lick away your tears. A dog's master is the center of their entire world and your sadness is a bit "contagious" when it comes to their existence.

In a study published in Animal Cognition, researchers even found that a dog was more likely to approach someone who is crying rather than someone humming or talking.

Your pet wants to soothe you when you're upset. In fact, dogs especially want to make everyone feel better.

There was a heartwarming story of a woman in an airport with a service Lab. The dog was new to his training and curled up next to a man who was silently crying while waiting for his plane. It was a beautiful way for that dog to help anyone in need.

Scientists aren't sure if dogs experience empathy as we do as humans, but this type of thing certainly supports that claim. I do know that dogs can identify sadness as something that is different than other feelings.

Allow your pet to soothe you. It's also helpful to get out of your funk by playing with your pet or taking them on a walk. It's a good way to put a little happy back into both of your worlds.

ME: TOTALLY STRESSED!

As a young veterinary student, I had a police officer walk into the hospital in the middle of the night with a 120-pound German shepherd police dog. Students are assigned cases, but during emergencies, it is first come, first serve. And I was up next.

The dog had broken his large canine tooth and was bleeding from his mouth.

There I was at 110 pounds with this 120-pound dog who was certainly bigger than me. The nice six feet five, 280 pound police officer with his ginormous dog made me look like a toddler.

"What is the dog's name?" I asked after he brought his animal (who was in pain) into an exam room.

"His name is Sid," said the officer. "And I need to tell you upfront that he is a trained and dangerous police dog. I will tell you how to handle him and you will be perfectly fine."

Perfectly fine. Yes, I would be…if I weren't eaten.

"How do I go about becoming perfectly fine?" I asked.

"If you put Sid into a kennel, he's going to attack the kennel until you give him the release to not attack it," the officer explained. "You need to say, 'Off. Set. Go' when you want him to stand down – and he will listen to you."

"You cannot be afraid," he warned. "He smells fear."

Not be afraid of the dangerous police dog that was bigger than me...no problem!

Yes, I was afraid as I brought Sid back to the kennels, but I decided to listen to the officer and do exactly what he told me.

I wondered: Would Sid even go into one of the kennels without whipping around and launching an attack on me? I kept practicing those words in my mind: Off. Set. Go. Off. Set. Go. That was the code...for survival.

As I maneuvered him back to the bigger kennels and leaned down to open the door, Sid and I were eye-to-eye. I could tell he was tensing up, so I said the magic words: "Off. Set. Go." Sid calmly stepped into the kennel. When I closed the door, he began to attack it. I said the words again, "Off. Set. Go." Sid stopped on a dime and immediately laid down.

He was happy, chilled out and seemed to read the look on my face, which was saying, "Please don't kill me. I'm not afraid...really."

Sid was just as easy to deal with as I took him out of the kennel and brought him to his procedure. Of course, I told everyone around the magic code although they insisted I stick around since I was the Sid Whisperer.

I love this story because it shows just how quickly we can de-stress and mellow out our animals if they are and we are trained properly.

9

Common Sense From The Conscious Vet

When I had children, it was a rocky beginning. I had raised countless pets, but I had never raised a human. Pets are dependent on you, but they mature rather quickly and I feel that they are not so delicate as baby humans. These small beings taught me many valuable lessons. When I didn't know what to do with babies, I thought to myself, "What would I do with my dog?" Quite often, I would have an answer.

When I would accidently step on our small Chihuahua in the kitchen I wouldn't make a big deal out of it (luckily it was never a big deal), but I would tell her, "You're okay. Keep a positive attitude. You're not really hurt." Luckily, she was fine. It was the same for my toddlers who fell down and upon first sniff, I'd say, "Get up. You got this. Keep going."

With people and pets, if you keep a positive attitude and not make it a dramatic experience then you can actually teach resilience, capability and confidence.

Our existence with one another as humans is very similar to how animals operate—we, just make it more complicated because we think a little too hard sometimes. What helped me get through raising my three girls was to keep it as simple as possible, reward behaviors I wanted, and create a connection that is unbreakable through love and kindness.

My first-born presented many challenges and obstacles. She cried unless I was holding her and she was quite affected by certain foods that I ate because I was breastfeeding. Dairy caused her to projectile vomit and orange juice caused her to cry in pain most of the day. I quickly learned how food affected the body. I became an avid label reader as my daughter grew up, as I had to avoid all dairy products and I suddenly realized it seemed as if everything had dairy in it!

As I was reading labels I noticed how many dyes, preservatives, salt and words I couldn't pronounce were in our foods. I started applying this knowledge to pet foods and figured out many of the same issues. Pet foods were filled with junk, highly processed and many had additives and preservatives.

I then started to think about all the exotic species that I vetted. These species required specialized diets, most of which were either fed raw or prepared foods by their owners. For example, bearded dragons eat crickets, worms and fresh dark leafy greens in addition to other calcium rich vegetables. All of this was fresh and if this fresh diet and the right environment were provided to the dragon, he would not get sick.

I started to apply this to cats and dogs. If they eat more fresh food and I provide the right environment for the animal to thrive, there will be less illness. I started recommending grain-free minimally processed, naturally preserved with no additives and dyes type foods to my clients. Cats and dogs lost weight, skin problems, ear infections, upset stomachs and urinary issues started to clear up. This was fascinating to me. I soon realized the importance of what you put in your pet is what you get out.

It is much the same with children and people. If you put junk in, you get junk out. But if you provide your pet or yourself with minimally processed real healthy foods with the correct environment, you stay overall healthy.

Common Sense Tip #1: Feed high quality raw or minimally processed food with no dyes, no synthetic preservatives and no additives to your pet. Be able to pronounce the ingredient list. Educate yourself on what is healthy food and what is recommended for the species you have.

A word of caution, if you decide to feed a raw diet: Please do not feed raw meat from the grocery store. This is meat that is meant to be cooked. There are high quality commercially prepared safe raw pet food diets, be sure to do your research.

Common Sense Tip #2: In addition to quality food, staying lean via exercising is crucial. Lean pets that are exercised live longer. Period. The benefits of exercise for your pets are endless: It releases natural endorphins that make them feel better; it strengthens muscle and bone; it reduces weight; it can increase their energy level; it helps the skin health; it helps memory and brain health; and it also helps with relaxation and good quality sleep. It is even known to prevent cancer. Keep them lean and exercise them. Even better, exercise with your pet. You will reap the same benefits. A brisk walk with your dog will reward both of you.

Common Sense Tip #3: Pets Hide Illness. Most of our pets are relatively small, smaller than us (yes, there are exceptions). As a general rule, animals hide disease. I talked earlier how pets use their instincts. If they look sick, guess what happens in the wild? They get eaten. So, until they are really sick, they don't always show the outward signs.

Pets are certainly not like people in this regard. We typically complain about our stuffed-up nose, our headache and that our back hurts. Pets do not moan about it. Pets normally look good unless something is really wrong. A dog that does not greet you at the door when he normally does, a bird at the bottom of the cage not perching or singing, a cat that hides in the closet and never has gone in there; these are all signs of illness in a pet. When pets are ill, they like to separate from the pack. They do this so they do not make the pack vulnerable to being attacked. Now, I know your pet's pack is you and your family members, but if your pet is hiding, it is telling you something.

The small size of most of our pets combined with hiding behaviors requires a vet visit. Certain pets like rabbits, guinea pigs and birds can die suddenly if some conditions are not tended to quickly. They are also quite small, so not eating and not drinking can make them head south fast. Small pets become dehydrated quickly especially if they are experiencing diarrhea or vomiting.

If any pet is vomiting, do not try to feed it right away. Think about it. If you just vomited would you want to eat or drink? No way. You need your belly to rest, and if doesn't get better then consider seeking medical attention. If it does feel better in a couple of hours perhaps then you will try small sips of liquid to see how they do. If dogs and cats vomit, let their bellies rest for several hours before offering food or water. If the vomiting continues, seek medical attention.

Common Sense Tip #4: Preventative Care Is Cheaper Than Sick Care. At my hospitals, we stress preventative care so you come in once a year to see me instead of several sick visits. Feeding the right foods, getting exercise and keeping your pet lean is a great place to start. Having annual preventative care exams with laboratory tests like fecal exams and blood tests, are also essential. As a veterinarian, I can look at the outside of your pet and determine if it is healthy, but I cannot see into your pet so testing bloodwork, urine and fecal samples sometimes are necessary. This is how you find disease before it makes your pet sick.

Testing fecal samples twice yearly on your pet is important, especially dogs. Think about it, your dog goes outside barefoot 365 days per year then comes inside, licks his private areas and his feet. When you really think about it, it is rather gross. Wherever he walks he can pick up things like intestinal parasites which linger on his feet. He licks his paws and ingests them.

The same goes for our indoor cats. They may not go outside, but we do. We walk in with our shoes and our cats walk barefoot in house and clean their feet daily. It is very easy to see why we recommend checking fecal samples to catch things early. If your dog or cat does get an intestinal parasite, it is contagious to you.

Intestinal parasites are very common in our pets, especially those that are not on monthly heartworm prevention. Your pet can pass these intestinal parasites to you if you ingest any feces. Now that is really gross and I am sure you're thinking, "I would never eat my dog's poop!" I am sure you would not do this, but your dog licks the poop off of his bum and then licks you. If he hits your mouth, he could transfer those microscopic parasites to you. Over 150 children die every year of roundworm ingestion and then migration. Roundworms are a common intestinal parasite in our pets and are completely preventable with monthly deworming.

Common Sense Tip #5: Pet Connections Are Real and Valuable to Happiness and Well-Being. Studies have shown that one thing that keeps humans happy is connectedness. In Marci Shimoff's book, *Happy for No Reason*, she discusses how our connections with other humans are crucial for us to be happy. I would agree. To bring this further, I'd say that our connections with our pets can bring that same happiness into our lives. Pets show us love and kindness all the time; it's always up for offering.

Unlike our people connections, our pet connections give us the unconditional love and lack of judgement we seek from our human friends and family that may not always be there. I eavesdrop on my children (because I am a mom), and often they are having a conversation with our pets. Of course, it sounds one-sided but typically the net-net is my daughter is "figuring it out" on her own with support from a non-judgmental furry or scaly friend.

Common Sense Tip #6: Work Hard to Get What You Want. Have you ever seen a dog chase a squirrel up a tree and then sit under that tree for hours waiting for that squirrel to come down? Now you may not call that smart because if the dog is below the tree, the squirrel isn't coming down, but from the standpoint of tenacity, that dog has most of us beat. Call it a gut feeling, an instinct, a hopeful vision -- call it what you want -- but the dog is certain he is going to get the squirrel.

Be sure to go with your own gut when it comes to your decisions and your pet's decision. If something doesn't feel right, ask. If you are not getting the answers you want, find someone else. I always encourage my clients to get second opinions if they don't think I am right. The world is filled with many experts and the universe directs us to where our answers may lie. Don't take the answer if something in your gut isn't sitting right.

Common Sense Tip #7: Helping Your Pet Pass Is A Selfless and Loving Act. How do I know when its time to euthanize my pet? The answer: You just know. I have this discussion on a weekly basis with clients. I have many clients that tell me, "I don't want to play God, I can't make that decision." In the same breath they say, "I do not want my pet to suffer. How do I know?"

From my 20-plus years of experience in this field, I have learned this: When pets are really ill, they stop eating and drinking (most), they hide in places or lay in places they typically would not, and they try to separate from the pack. You are your pet's pack. Pets are selfless in this area. They don't want to make the pack vulnerable to disease or attack, so they separate and make themselves weak so it will be ended suddenly. Think about it, if your pet was in the wild and very debilitated and felt it was going to die, it would give up, so something stronger would end it soon to stop the pain and the suffering. No one, including our pets, want to suffer a slow and painful death.

Deciding to have your pet euthanized is a caring, altruistic act of kindness and love. Watch for these signs if you think your pet is suffering: They are being reclusive, not eating, not drinking, and not participating in life as they did before, perhaps they are laying in new spots which are very out of character. Listen to your gut. Sometimes, I have clients who tell me, "I can just tell she is suffering; it's not fair to prolong this."

That is very true. When you know the animal is suffering, we are fortunate to be able to have the decision option. Be sure to talk to your vet about these decisions.

We are here to guide you.

10

Miracle Stories

Healing animals is not just a job for me. It's the joy of my life. Years of vet school, plus many more in my practice, makes me a person who relies on the laws of science and medicine to help cure our companions.

I do like to leave a little room for the unexpected.

As I end my first book, I wanted to share with you a few of the miracle stories that touched my heart.

When a client walks through my door with something simple (or so it seems to them) like a swollen lymph node or a dog that is a little off his food, most of the time I find something simple to treat. Maybe it's just an infection or the dog has just a simple upset stomach. Sometimes, sadly, I find big, bad, horrible disease.

This is really the terrible part of my job … delivering devastating news to those who least expect it. Sometimes the news is inoperable cancer or maybe it's a condition that has no known treatments that work. Whatever the diagnosis, I will tell my owners not to tell their pets.

As crazy as it sounds, knowing you have a disease makes it worse. Our pets often do not know they are sick. We are the ones who label it, filling the situation with emotional distress and fear that we may lose our beloved pet.

There can be hope in what might seem like the worst possible times.

Over the past twenty years, I have been able to experience what I call the true miracles of pets. I have learned that nothing is impossible.

These stories prove that pets teach us love, how to slow down, how to be conscious and be present in the moment. They also teach us how to believe in miracles.

Writing them brought a few tears to my eyes (again).

THE BULL MASTIFF

I had been seeing Rocky's owners for several years. They were a young married couple that adored their dog and took impeccable care of him. Their beloved Bull Mastiff was their child. He was a giant breed dog with just as big a heart. The general rule is the bigger the dog, the shorter the lifespan. Many Bull Mastiffs don't even live to eight or nine years.

Rocky was nine and he had been limping for several weeks. They had tried to rest him but the limp was getting worse. I examined Rocky and the pain he experienced when I pushed on his hock (the ankle) made Rocky yelp! Giant breed dogs are particularly stoic, so I knew Rocky was in significant pain. We took X-rays of Rocky's leg and quite sadly, I discovered that Rocky's right hind leg was very abnormal. The bone was breaking down and there were substantial changes that were most consistent with bone cancer. Bone cancer is a terrible diagnosis in it of itself, but having bone cancer in a giant breed dog is even worse. Most of the time the treatment for bone cancer is leg amputation but removing a leg on such a heavy muscled breed can really cause some problems with mobility in these giant types.

I delivered the news to Rocky's parents and their hearts sank. They never thought a simple limp would end up being a possibility of an aggressive bone tumor. We discussed getting a definitive diagnosis, which would involve a bone biopsy. Rocky's owners agreed. I performed a biopsy and about a week later the results were in: Rocky had osteosarcoma, an aggressive malignant bone cancer. His owners were crushed. Their worst nightmare had come true.

After a couple of days to think about the diagnosis, it was important to Rocky's Mom and Dad to know all of their options, so I sent them to a veterinary oncologist for a consultation. Upon looking at the records, the oncologist noticed that the cancer crossed the joint. Osteosarcoma does not typically behave this way, so he recommended another biopsy to make sure the diagnosis was correct. The oncologist performed the second biopsy and it came back as malignant osteosarcoma again.

The owners were devastated. They had a small glimmer of hope only to find out their worst nightmare was confirmed, again.

Amputation of the leg and chemotherapy was the recommended route by the oncologist for the best survival, but the couple decided not to pursue this because Rocky was already nine years old. They were concerned for his mobility and his overall quality of life if this was such an aggressive bone tumor. Plus, they didn't want to put him through surgery and repeated medication injections if it was only going to buy them just six short months. They wanted his quality of life to be better and more peaceful. Rocky hated riding in the car and they knew this would entail multiple doctor visits. Instead, they opted to give him pain medications to keep him as comfortable as possible and lots more attention to make him feel happy and loved.

Several weeks later, the dog was far more than merely comfortable. He was running around their yard like a pup. "Doctor, it's really strange. He seems to have a new lease on life," said the owner. "He doesn't even limp anymore. The pain medicine really works well." I was so glad to hear this because Rocky had been in such pain. I was elated to see the medicine was working so well to keep him comfortable.

I did not see Rocky for another six months, which is when he came in limping again. This time he was acting very sick and would not even eat. He was very depressed, running a fever, and couldn't lift his head off the floor.

The owners were concerned it may be time. It had been six months and the oncologist had said they would be lucky to get two months with just pain medicine. Osteosarcoma is a malignant cancer that can spread anywhere in the body including the lungs and other organs. They were told when bone cancer spreads, it will make Rocky very, very sick.

I repeated the X-rays of his right hind leg and his lungs, plus took blood tests. The technician called me in to look at the X-ray.

It was normal.

This was very surprising. I re-read through my notes, the oncologist's notes and previous X-ray notes. The cancer was in the right hind leg. I double-checked with my technician that he had X-rayed the right hind limb and he did. I even had him repeat the X-ray in front of me because I couldn't believe my eyes! Much to my surprise, there was no evidence of cancer on the X-ray because the leg was normal. In fact, there was no sign of cancer on any of Rocky's X-rays or his blood tests.

So why was Rocky so sick? I continued to look for answers and tested Rocky for tick-borne disease. In New England, we have a lot of ticks and these ticks carry terrible disease and can make dogs very sick. Rocky tested positive for a tick-borne disease called Anaplasmosis. I treated Rocky immediately with IV fluids, antibiotics and pain medicine.

Rocky improved in two days and made a dramatic recovery from his Anaplasmosis infection. He lived for three more years and passed away at age 12, cancer free.

When I diagnose cancer in pets, I always tell the owner, "Don't tell your pet. He doesn't know and doesn't need to know."

I believe Rocky healed his cancer. I am not exactly sure how, but I think about it often and discuss these miracle cancer cures with my owners. I do not have the exact answer, but I am certain loving and caring owners with the right emotional vibes played a role.

A quick aside: Anita Moorjani is a cancer survivor that has written several books including *Dying To Be Me.* She tells of her journey from cancer to near death to healing her lymphoma. It is a miraculous book that talks about how to choose love over fear and to look for magnificence within yourself and others. I cannot explain to you as eloquently how Rocky healed his cancer as Anita gave her account of how she healed herself. What I can tell you is that I had the honor of meeting Anita and her authenticity, self-awareness, and beautiful aura were pure and fearless.

By the way, I don't know if animals in the wild die of terrible cancers or not. No one can tell us, but I believe that our pets try to live a pure life of who they are and we need to allow them to do it.

We need to allow ourselves to do the same.

THE GUINEA PIG

Oreo was an adorable black and white guinea pig. He looked like a Hampshire pig—black all over with a white stripe over his shoulders. I used to show Hampshire pigs at the fair when I was a child and I named them all Oreo, so this little guinea pig had a special place in my heart.

Oreo's owner rushed him to my hospital because she was certain he was dying. Oreo was lying on his side, breathing heavy and his belly was enlarged and very painful. I quickly gave Oreo pain medicine to make him feel more comfortable and I immediately took X-rays. Oreo's stomach was severely distended with air. He had a life-threatening condition called bloat. This is a condition where the stomach fills with air and presses on the largest vessel (vena cava) in the body and it decreases blood flow to the heart. Many guinea pigs that have bloat do not survive.

I had the task of telling the owner the news and she began to cry. "If he's not going to make it, I want to take him home," she said. "I want to do everything possible for Oreo to keep him comfortable."

There were many treatments I could do in hopes that Oreo would beat the odds. I gave him multiple injections, fluids, pain medicine, and detailed instructions so the owner could keep him as comfortable as possible. I showed the owner how to hand feed Oreo, massage his belly, and instructed her to pick up additional medicine at the drug store to help with the gas.

The owner took Oreo back home and was hopeful he would make it through the night or at least the medicines would allow him a comfortable passing. I waited for the phone call the next morning to tell me Oreo's fate. I got a phone call from his happy owner who told me that the Oreo was running around his cage and eating on his own. I asked her to bring him in for X-rays, and the bloat was gone.

I now tell owners a different prognosis with this condition. With medicine and treatments all night long, some guinea pigs will survive.

Oreo did.

THE OLDEST CAT

Remember in a previous chapter, I discussed how my number one tip for keeping your pets healthy for a long, long time is that you keep them lean and exercised? You also have to trust in the judgment of the right vet in order to help them. The oldest cat in my practice was Elvis, a medium haired orange tiger cat and he lived to be 25-years-old. When Elvis was 22, he started eating a lot and losing a lot of weight. After laboratory tests, I found that Elvis had an overactive thyroid gland.

There were several options for Elvis to treat his overactive thyroid including daily medicine, radioactive iodine treatment or surgery. After careful consideration by Elvis's owner, they asked me to do surgery. I wasn't exactly excited to perform surgery on a 22-year old cat, in fact, I was very concerned he may not make it through the anesthesia. As a doctor, I know age isn't a disease but I had never performed surgery on such an elderly patient.

Elvis was an outdoor kitty and sometimes he would be out hunting, so giving medicine two times a day was out of the question. The radioactive iodine treatment would require him to be in the hospital almost a week and the owners thought he would not do well being caged for long since he has known so much freedom. Surgery, a day procedure, seemed the best way to treat Elvis.

The day of the surgery was a bit nerve racking for everyone. The thought of anesthetizing a 22-year old cat made everyone more vigilant with every step. I knew this would be like anesthetizing a 150-year old human! Thankfully, the anesthesia, the surgery and the recovery were flawless. Elvis did amazing! In fact, he acted like nothing happened, and he certainly wanted to go home meowing. He reminded us the rest of the day as in: "Excuse me, I need to leave. Meow. Meow. Meow."

Elvis lived another three years as an outdoor cat. Besides his street-savvy-ness, his diet, lean body and being able to constantly exercise outside must have contributed to his longevity.

MY OWN DOG

My Basenji Toby lived to be 20. He not only had longevity, but he had tenacity. One of Toby's annoying habits was to chew up books when I wasn't paying attention. He was also very savvy at picking the books that would immediately grab my attention. He chewed many vet schoolbooks (which I used frequently) and when I had children, he chewed children's books, especially those that I read a lot. He chewed books until he was 19 years old.

When Toby was 17, I started to buy small bags of food because I thought he could die at any time. I am not sure why I started doing this, he was acting normal, and had no medical issues besides slowing down a bit. I just knew from my many other patients that a 17-year old dog is *old*! But Toby lived on.

He, along with Elvis, and many other older pets taught me that age is not a disease. Just because the number is high, it doesn't mean they are sick! It does however teach us what contributes to longevity. For Toby, he was exercised daily, he ate many fresh foods, he was lean, received great medical care and he had a family that loved him dearly.

I would clean and polish Toby's teeth every year until he was 17 and then I stopped. Again, not sure why I did this except I thought he was *old*. At age 19, I realized that his teeth were dreadful, his breath smelled terrible and his hair coat was dull and rough. I decided Toby needed his teeth cleaned so I anesthetized my 19-year old dog and cleaned his teeth.

He was a bit disoriented that evening after the procedure but the next few days were amazing. He had a new spring in his step and he felt significantly better. His hair coat improved because dogs clean themselves with their mouths and if the mouth is filled with bacteria and disease, it spreads to their hair coat.

After a few short weeks, he was almost like a puppy again. I really regretted not doing this sooner—I could have made him feel better well before he was 19.

Toby and Elvis taught me a lot about the age of a pet—it doesn't matter. Disease matters. Old healthy pets can do the same things as young healthy pets; they just have a different number label, that's all. Lean and exercised animals live the longest, but having that loving home also makes a difference.

I am pretty sure that if we look at people and longevity, we will find the same things.

TWO CATS. TWO CURES.

Cats truly do have nine lives. I believe that some of them live 16 lives because cats are magical in many ways and heal themselves. We can learn so much about resilience with cats.

One of the most common silent problems in domesticated cats is heart disease. There are typically no outward signs of heart disease until they are in heart failure. Heart failure is when the heart has a difficult time pumping and fluid backs up into or around their lungs making it incredibly difficult to breathe. Sadly, many cats will die if these signs are not recognized and they do not get medical help as soon as possible.

One little orange tabby, Marcus, came to see me on emergency with difficulty breathing and with his owners hysterically crying. Marcus had been the picture of health, but the past few days they noticed him sleeping a bit more than usual. They didn't think it was a big deal; they had had friends over from out of town, so they thought Marcus was just tired from all the new activity in the house.

I took X-rays of Marcus and his chest was full of fluid and that was why he could not breathe well—it was like he was drowning. I quickly was able to give Marcus medication, drain the fluid and placed Marcus on oxygen to manage his heart disease.

An hour later, the cat that was on death's door was practically a new feline. His face seemed to say, "Thanks – and can I leave now?" Marcus was purring, rubbing his whiskers and face on the oxygen tent and doing what I call "making muffins," which is kneading his paws into the cushy bed in his oxygen cage. He was visibly happy.

It's amazing how quickly cats respond to treatments and practically "fix themselves" in no time at all. I have been with people who have congestive heart failure and they are typically in the hospital for days to get stable. Not cats. Give them some medicine plus some oxygen and they are ready to go in hours. Quite amazing creatures!

Cats always astonish me with their ability to heal. One of my elderly clients who owned an older cat named Ralph called me one day in a panic saying that the always sweet and serene Ralph was hissing at her. "I think he wants to bite me," she said.

Ralph had never acted like this in the 12 years I had been treating him, so I reminded her that this wasn't normal behavior. I added that she should stay away from Ralph until we arrived. "He won't let you touch him. He won't let anyone go near him," she told me.

We did a house call where we somehow got a very upset Ralph into a carrier and brought him to the hospital. With the help of a little pain medicine and anesthesia, I was able to finally look at him. He had not one, but four abscessed teeth. Anyone – human or feline – would be in a very bad mood given those particulars.

I successfully removed the abscessed teeth and Ralph woke up. A few hours later, he was rubbing on the cage door and purring. He was instantly a happy kitty again and couldn't wait to be held by his happy owner. Ralph even went home the same day proving again that cats need very little recovery time.

I would like to add that when pets have really out of the ordinary behavior— please listen to this. They are typically trying to tell you something. This would not be the first time I have seen pets having a behavior problem that was a true medical problem stemming from pain or distress.

A LITTLE BIRD WITH A BIG WILL

A married couple that was beating the odds had a little parakeet that they deeply loved called Bird. The woman was in a wheel chair and had limited movements with her upper body; the man was physically challenged and had difficulty walking and doing simple movements. Because of this couples' physical limitations, I always made house calls for them because they were unable to drive to my hospital.

Bird was a very special pet to this couple. He would sit on their kitchen table and communicate "bird-talk" daily and became a loved member of their family. I was able to witness these three having full on conversations and Bird was part of all the discussions. Suddenly, Bird started to not talk as much and seemed to be breathing heavier than normal. I examined Bird and I discovered he had a huge mass growing on his body. It was on his lower abdomen and it was almost half the size of him. The owners felt terrible that they did not notice sooner. I explained that under the feathers, it is difficult to see, but I could feel it. Because of the owner's physical limitations, they did not feel Bird ever. They could only look at him, so they felt terrible they had missed this very large mass.

These masses are not unusual for parakeets that are on all seed diets. They are typically fatty tumors that can grow very large, and eventually the bird can't move around anymore. In fact, it is not unusual for these tumors to grow half the size of the bird or even larger.

"Unfortunately, there's nothing I can do," I told them.

"Can't you do surgery," asked the young woman.

"Well, the bird is so small that there would be too much blood loss. He wouldn't make it through a surgery," I told her, sadly. "I can't do anything but you can. You can gradually change his diet from seed to more veggies and fruits, so you reduce the fat. You can make him as comfortable as possible by providing him with low perches and a handicapped cage so he will live out his life more easily."

She said, "I'm just going to love Bird a lot."

I agreed this was the best thing they could do.

Several months later, she called me and said, "Guess what? The mass just fell off."

"What?" I said.

"It fell off. It's at the bottom of the cage," she said. "Bird is alive and I found the mass on the bottom of his cage."

I will be honest. I didn't believe it. I made a special house call to see the couple and Bird because, frankly, I thought I was going to find something else. Masses just don't fall off.

I examined Bird and sure enough, this miracle animal was fine and without the mass. It was *gone*! I was looking at a perfectly healthy pet again. "Medically speaking, he walled it off. His little body knew this shouldn't be there and got rid of it, sort of like expelling a splinter because it doesn't belong," I explained to them. "The body has the ability to do that, which means that your Bird is fine."

"I told you," she said. "I just loved him and Bird got fixed. That's what happened."

I do believe that is what happened. I have no other explanation other than Bird healed himself with powers that are not visible to us. There are modalities of healing much greater than medicine and surgery. This level of energy healing isn't visible but it happens and I am thankful to be part of witnessing the impossible.

ONE LUCKY HOMING PIGEON

One of my favorite stories of all time revolves around a homing pigeon my staff named Charlotte, Charlotte Pendragon to be exact. Charlotte Pendragon was a famous female magician and Charlotte's story was exactly that magical.

On a beautiful spring day in our growing community, a strapping construction guy came into the hospital holding a little white thing in his hand. The man was covered in black asphalt because they were paving outside my hospital, but in his clean, heavy hands he gently cupped a little white pigeon. She was struggling on the side of the road, trying to fly, and he stopped his machine to rescue her.

The man wasn't sure what to do but he wanted us to assure him we would take good care of her. He even promised to stop by at the end of the day to check on the bird (and did!).

After examining Charlotte, I was concerned that her leg was broken and X-rays confirmed it. She had fractured her tibia, the bone in the lower part of the leg. I gave Charlotte pain medicine and anesthetized her while casting her small, delicate bone. During the procedure, we noticed that her legs were banded.

She was a homing pigeon.

Thank goodness for the Internet. My staff was not only Googling names for this pigeon but also looking up how to find the owner of a homing pigeon. He happened to live in Pennsylvania. My staff member called him, and as the story goes, there had been a homing pigeon race, but that day it stormed and poor Charlotte didn't return with the rest of the birds. It was not unusual for pigeons during a race to get off track, but they typically return a few days later. Now, it had been several days and the owner was very excited we had his Charlotte.

"I'll send you money," he said.

"The important thing," I said, "was how can I get your bird back to you."

He couldn't make the trip, but said not to worry about it.

"When the bird heals, you can release her and she will fly back to me. She will come home."

Charlotte was with me for eight weeks in the hospital and I grew very fond of the little bird. Each day, she became stronger and more full of personality. Naturally, I was a nervous wreck when I thought about releasing this little bird to fly home. How in the world would she get back to Pennsylvania after all of this time? She was in New Hampshire and we were several states away!

What if she was confused and got hurt again? She would be so vulnerable out there all alone.

When her leg was healed, we did a practice fly after hours and allowed her to let loose all over the inside of the animal hospital. She seemed to do a very good job taking flight in the hallways. A few weeks later and it was clear that this bird was perfectly strong and healthy.

It was time.

I was teary-eyed when we went outside on a beautiful summer's day. That moment of release was one of the most moving of my entire life. I felt the warm summer breeze, opened my hands and this trusting little bird flapped once, then twice, and took flight.

Charlotte seemed to know that it would be fine. She began to soar higher and higher and then faster and farther until I couldn't see her anymore.

I couldn't wait for time to pass and to make that phone call.

"Yes, I have her here with me now," said the happy owner.

Charlotte was home, which proved that animals do find me. But many times, I have to let them go.

11

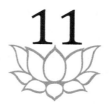

Saying Goodbye

I don't think there has been a week where a client did not say, "The hardest part of your job must be to put a pet to sleep." My response is always the same.

"No, it is not. It is the greatest privilege to end pain and suffering."

I've had two people very close to me pass away of horrible, lingering deaths. One was my father-in-law, Len, a very loving man with a big heart. He was a former Chief in the military and had a tough side to him while he was also very practical. Len had a multitude of medical issues stemming from smoking for 50 years. He had congestive heart failure compounded by emphysema, so breathing was very difficult. He was on oxygen 24-7 and I forgot to mention, he also had diabetes. He handled these diseases in stride and never complained.

As the diseases became worse, his kidneys started to fail. When the kidneys fail, the body slowly shuts down, you don't want to eat, you retain fluid, you don't urinate and you start to hallucinate. He didn't know his son or his wife. It took nine grueling days of no eating, no drinking, constant nausea and finally he slipped into a coma. I can only hope at this point, he felt no pain.

My mother suffered the same injustices of human medical conditions while in the care of a hospital. She had colon cancer and it had spread, and she threw a large clot that cut the circulation off to the lower half her body. While her feet, her ankles, the lower part of her legs, then her thighs turned black from lack of circulation, she was pumped full of fentanyl in hopes she would endure the pain of her lower body dying. They covered her legs tightly with blankets, so I would not notice her limbs turning black from death.

My mother was a strong woman who never complained of any pain though she suffered from headaches her whole life. While she lay in her hospital bed she moaned and cried, I could only believe the pain of impending death was too much to bear.

Human medicine is cruel. I would never, could never allow this to happen to a cat, a dog or any little creature. I could lose my license if I let a pet suffer unduly. It is considered abuse.

I consider humane euthanasia a gift. Euthanasia means good death. Our pets are fortunate. If they are suffering and there is no more we can do, we can peacefully end their distress. As a veterinarian, we are allowed this gift to give.

Molly was a small black cat with brilliant green eyes. Her owners loved her dearly and she was the only pet and the first pet they ever had together. Molly developed a tumor in her ear that was inoperable and the cancer had spread to her lungs. She was no longer eating and the side of her face would wince and twitch. The owners felt the pain medicine was no longer helping her and they wanted to help her pass.

Both mom and dad brought Molly to my hospital on her last day. Molly was a very fidgety cat who never wanted to sit still. Her mom longed for her to just sit in her lap while I delivered the medicine through her IV to end her hardship with this tumor in her ear. My technicians had placed an IV catheter in her front leg and mom was holding her tight next to her chest. What happened next was astonishing.

As Molly fidgeted in mom's arms, mom started to chant a Native American Indian chant. Molly settled. Mom continued the call. I do not remember the words, but I do remember the energy and how this chant resonated with me.

It was complete peace.

Molly settled more in Mom's arms and looked up toward the ceiling. This was a cat that never sat still and I had not sedated her, but this chant calmed Molly (and everyone in the room). And then I delivered her medicine through her IV.

Molly passed peacefully.

Mom and dad sat holding their beloved cat. Mom slowed her chant then stopped. It may have been one of the most beautiful passings I have ever witnessed.

It is true that the hardest thing is saying goodbye to a loving pet. It doesn't matter if they have been in your life a few days or a few decades. That pet has made an important and unforgettable mark in your life.

I still think about all of my beloved animals and dream of the day when I can see all of them again. However, if you pay attention, our pets only leave us in body, not in spirit.

Buster was one of the most obnoxious dogs at my hospital. He barked incessantly while he sat with his owner in the exam room. His owner, an older woman with a heart of gold, would take treat bags that we had for sale off the shelf and feed them to Buster to get him to stop barking. What mom was doing was encouraging the behavior so every time Buster came to the hospital, he would bark and mom would buy another bag of treats or maybe even two bags to keep Buster quiet.

Buster may have been an obnoxious barker, but his smile and tail wag warmed your heart. He was 80 pounds of love and tenderness. He lived to be 16 years old, which is very unusual for a large breed dog.

On the day of Buster's passing, mom came to my hospital and she was in Exam Room 1. This was the exam room we typically put Buster in because it was the biggest for a large dog. This time was different. Buster wasn't barking; there were no treats. Buster was very ill. I sat with mom while she said her good-byes and we discussed Buster's long life and how he could no longer hang on. It was time.

Again, my technicians had placed an IV catheter in Buster's leg, so I had access to a vein and I delivered the medicine through the IV to allow Buster to pass peacefully.

In a few minutes, Buster no longer had any pain. He had passed. Mom made jokes about how he barked non-stop when he would come to the hospital. We laughed. We both stood up and Mom was about to leave the room. Both our backs were to Buster as he lay peacefully on the exam room floor. Then, out of nowhere, BANG! a bag of treats hit the floor! It had fallen off the shelf. Both mom and I looked back and saw the bag of treats by her beloved dog. I looked at Mom and said, "Buster is telling you good-bye…and that you forgot his treats!"

Mom smiled and we both laughed.

Our pets never leave us.

Be sure to watch for the signs.

AN EUTHANSIA DECISION

Making an euthanasia decision is very difficult. I know and understand the struggle in each client's heart. Most clients want to make sure of two things: Their pet is not suffering and they are not keeping the animal alive for them.

An older couple owned Chloe, a dilute Calico cat, that was slowly going off her food and not playing as much anymore. Chloe had always been a very active cat with a bit of spitfire to her.

That seemed to be fading for her.

Upon exam, I noted that Chloe was breathing very heavy. After we had taken X-rays, I discovered her chest was full of fluid. When fluid surrounds the lungs, cats do not function well and it feels like a drowning sensation.

Fluid in the chest can mean many things. After I tested Chloe's chest fluid, I found out that it was cancer. Cancer in the lungs is a devastating diagnosis, but there were a few things we could do. We were able to remove the fluid from her chest and make her comfortable for several months.

Mom and Dad wanted the absolute best for Chloe and did not want her to suffer at all. We discussed that chemotherapy was not an option for this cancer and made a plan. When Chloe exhibited any signs of distress, they would elect euthanasia.

The day arrived. Chloe's respirations were difficult and she had stopped eating the day prior. She was no longer greeting them at the door and was hiding in the closet. She had also settled into a strong abnormal purr. They were certain it was time for Chloe to pass, but their love for their cat was strong and thought of losing her was overwhelming.

"Are we doing the right thing?" Mom asked me. "I do not want her to suffer, but I don't want to keep her alive just for me."

I assured Mom and Dad that they wouldn't be there asking if they didn't know that the time was right. Though it is so difficult to do, accepting that the time you pick is the right time is the right thing. Not allowing your pet to suffer and giving them a peaceful passing is a selfless act of kindness and gift of love.

Chloe passed in Mom's loving arms.

After they spent time, I carried Chloe away. They kissed her head and gave her one last stroke across her silky fur.

"We did the right thing," Mom said through her tears.

"Yes, you did. She is at peace now and you did the right thing," I agreed.

Letting a pet go is painful and incredibly difficult, but trust the time is right and the decision is filled with grace.

I'm asked again and again about when is it time to get a new pet? That depends on you. When the time is right, you will feel it and know when there is a spot in your heart to be filled.

I always think of the story of Gemini, a long-haired feisty black cat who lived with a retired soldier who had served in the Iraq war. Nineteen-year-old Gemini was this soldier's rock, her reason to get up in the morning, her reason to get through her day and her reason why she knew love in her heart. This cat was adored. Gemini lived a long and beautiful life. After she passed, it was a very difficult time for the soldier who didn't know if she could ever love another feline again.

"No one could ever replace Gemini," she cried.

"No one ever will," I assured her. "But certainly, there is another pet out there who will benefit from your love and care. Gemini would want you to have another friend."

She finally made the decision to get a pet and wanted a Chinese Crested hairless dog. To find one required a road trip across country to Indiana where there was a breeder. The soldier and her partner drove there and both were quite stressed about it. She still felt she was "replacing" Gemini and great guilt was in her heart.

They agreed to meet the breeder at her store in a quaint downtown area of rural America. The store was named....you'll never believe it. Gemini's. "I know we're doing the right thing," the solider said to her partner.

A little Chinese Crested named Gracie Mae entered their life that day and now she runs the show. She's six, beautiful and the second love of this soldier's life. Gracie is not a replacement. She's just someone else this soldier was meant to have in her heart.

There is a lot of room in one heart.

The connection you had with the pet that passed will never be replaced. The lessons you learned from that animal are unique and will last you a lifetime. But you've already learned those lessons. You might even long for the same connection, but it will never happen.

Each lesson is to be learned.

Each dog, cat or animal is with you for a different reason.

Each period of time with your pet is priceless.

Every connection you make is pure animality.

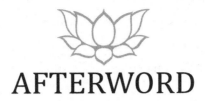

AFTERWORD

Thank you for taking the time to read my first book. I hope to write several others where we can examine the unique world of animals and their care.

It's a topic that endlessly fascinates me because if I know one thing about the animals in our lives, it's this wonderful given: The unconditional love from animal to person is pure, raw and real. Animals bring out the love and kindness in humans, which are two traits that we often lose in such a fast-moving society.

The other day I watched my own cats. One was very sick and the other sat on the floor next to him licking his head to make him feel better. That's love on a very primal level. How many times have you walked in after a bad day and just one lick from your pet made it so much better? It's so basic and beautiful, so simple and so complex.

Pets meet us, trust us and then turn on that love.

It's a joy to watch, an honor to be part of their world.

Animals are a good reminder to us as humans to be a little kinder to people and other animals in the world. Why? I believe that animals are big teachers of karma. What you put out is what you get back. The thing with animals is they give us everything and I hope that they get back the love they need and deserve. One of my favorite sayings is: I hope I can be as great as my pet thinks I am.

Bottom line: Our pets provide us with spiritual, physiological, psychological, and emotional fulfillment that create a much larger experience when pulled together than one can imagine when they hold that guinea pig, puppy or cat for the first time.

Animals love from such a pure place. Their love isn't passive aggressive. It doesn't have a catch. There is no "you do this and I'll do that." It's not conditional. An animal never thinks, I like you because…..

They just think, "I like you because I like you."

Until next time,

Melissa

Please visit my Facebook page Dr. Melissa Magnuson, The Conscious Vet

Acknowledgements

It takes a village and I thank you all:

To my clients who provided me with endless joy, stories and lessons. I thank you for choosing me as your veterinarian and sharing your priceless possessions with me.

To my husband and girls who provide me with unconditional love, support, respect and understanding of long workdays and a career that cannot shut off. I love you more.

To my most awesome staff (and Lisa) that supports my limitless energy and ideas: you are all gifts.

To my mom and dad, who raised me to be incredibly responsible, have an undying work ethic, and provided me with a childhood of character building experiences, I thank you.

To my sister (and her family), for listening and thinking every story I have ever told was wonderful, your ears are gold.

To Danielle MacKinnon, John Holland and Julie Stockbridge for opening my eyes to my intuitive side and learning about psychic abilities.

To Cindy Pearlman for her writing artistry.

To Peter Hartel for your gifted drawing talent.

To Mrs. Olson for always asking when my book was going to be done. It kept me on track and made me smile.